Abdelhamid H. Elgazzar

A Concise Guide
to Nuclear Medicine

Foreword by

Henry N. Wagner, Jr., M.D

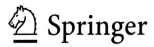 Springer

Author

Abdelhamid H. Elgazzar, MD., FCAP
Diplomate, American Board of Nuclear Medicine
Diplomate, American Board of Pathology
Professor and Chairman
Department of Nuclear Medicine, Kuwait University
Chairman, Faculty of Nuclear Medicine
Kuwait Institute of Medical Specializations
Chairman, Council of Nuclear Medicine
Ministry of Health, Kuwait
Safat 13110
Kuwait
aelgazzar49@hotmail.com

ISBN 978-3-642-19425-2   e-ISBN 978-3-642-19426-9
DOI 10.1007/978-3-642-19426-9
Springer Heidelberg Dordrecht London New York

Library of Congress Control Number: 2011925945

Cover design: eStudioCalamar, Figueres/Berlin

Printed on acid-free paper

Springer is part of Springer Science+Business Media (www.springer.com)

To

My friends who selflessly supported over the years

Foreword

In France in 1896, Henri Becquerel discovered that certain materials emitted energetic "rays," later called radioactive decay. In 1929, American physicist Ernest Lawrence built the first cyclotron and was able to produce positron-emitting radionuclides. In 1931, Dirac postulated the existence of the positron as an antiparticle having the same mass as an electron but with a positive rather than negative charge. The proof of the existence of the positrons was proved in cosmic radiation by another Nobel Prize winner, Carl Anderson, in 1932. That same year French physicists Irene Curie (daughter of Marie Curie) and Frederick Joliot (Irene's husband) announced their discovery of artificial radioactivity. They showed that many different atoms could be made radioactive. With the Curie/Joliot publication, Lawrence immediately recognized the enormous potential value of being able to make "radioactive tracers" that made possible medically important as well as chemical and physical measurements. Subsequent pioneers recognized the great biological importance of the radioactive elements that a cyclotron could produce, including oxygen-15 and carbon-11. In the spring of 1945, the US government made the decision to produce radioisotopes for civilian use. In June 1946, President Truman signed an executive order that made iodine-131 available from Oak Ridge National Laboratory to qualified physicians throughout the United States. The first shipment of carbon-14 was on August 2, 1946, to Martin Kamen at Berkeley, California. The shipment was kept secret because Kamen was falsely thought at the time to be a communist. The first announced shipment to a civilian institution was subsequently to the Barnard Free Skin and Cancer Hospital at Washington University in St. Louis. On December 7, 1946, the revolutionary announcement was made by an internist, Sam Seidlin and colleagues, that radioiodine could not just ameliorate but cure metastatic cancer. According to Marshall Brucer at Oak Ridge, within days, every Congressman had heard from his constituency, and on January 1, 1947, the Atomic Energy Commission (AEC) took over the distribution of radioisotopes from the supersecret Manhattan District Project of World War II that had developed the atomic bomb.

In 1946, George Moore, a neurosurgeon at the University of Minnesota, used iodine-131 labeled iodofluorescein to localize brain tumors using a Geiger–Muller detector in 12 patients during surgery. In 1950, the FDA recognized iodine-131 as the first "radioactive new drug." The public was excited by news of the use of radioiodine not only in the diagnosis of hypo- and hyperthyroidism but in the treatment of thyroid diseases as well in many patients, eliminating the need for surgery. It was the first example of defining disease on the basis of a measured regional molecular process, that is, the accumulation of radioactive iodine.

"Radioisotope scanning" was the name given to imaging of the distribution of radioactive tracers in the living human body at various times after injection of a radioactive "tracer." New "radiopharmaceuticals" were developed as a means of "visualizing" previously invisible organs, such as the liver, that could not be examined effectively by conventional x-rays.

Clinical molecular imaging is about uncovering physiology noninvasively by probing specific cellular and molecular processes in vivo. What has made molecular imaging so exciting now is the introduction of efficient, high-sensitivity devices for preclinical (animal model) as well as clinical imaging. Hybrid imaging devices, which combine the high resolution of anatomic imaging with the physiologic techniques, have become widespread in clinical practice and enable determination of a metabolic or receptor defect with pinpoint accuracy within minutes. Molecular imaging is now widely used throughout the world to detect disease, and to plan and evaluate the success of treatment.

Oncology has been the most fruitful domain of molecular imaging at present, particularly because of the information provided in measuring the energy supply of lesions, the abundance of unexploited tumor markers and intra- and intercellular communication pathways amenable to imaging.

This useful book describes how molecular imaging is used to answer the questions raised in the practice of medicine: (1) What is the patient's problem? (2) Where is the problem? (3) What is going to happen? (4) What is the best course of action ? (5) Is the treatment effective? Medicine has moved from whole body to organs to tissues to cells and now to molecules. We are indeed in a revolutionary time in the history of medicine, and it behooves all medical students and physicians to learn how to use this revolutionary approach to diagnose disease, plan, and monitor treatment.

Henry N. Wagner, Jr., MD

Preface

Nuclear medicine utilizes radioactive molecules (radiopharmaceuticals) for the diagnosis and treatment of disease. The diagnostic information obtained from imaging the distribution of radiopharmaceuticals is functional and thus fundamentally differs from other imaging techniques which are primarily anatomic in nature. The discipline of nuclear medicine uses highly advanced technology whose main emphasis in providing functional, rather than anatomical, information for patient management. Technological innovations are constantly adding more sophisticated imaging devices that provide impressive sensitivity and better resolution; hence nuclear medicine is a rapidly developing and changing field.

The idea behind this handbook is to acquaint students with the basic principles of nuclear medicine, the instrumentation used, the gamut of procedures available, and the judgments used to select specific diagnostic or therapeutic procedures and interpret results.

The book is for the students and professionals to: (a) be familiar with the common indications for nuclear medicine procedures, (b) understand the pathophysiologic basis of the common functional procedures, (c) understand the complementary role of diagnostic nuclear medicine in solving various clinical diagnostic problems, and (d) understand the basic principles of the therapeutic applications of nuclear medicine.

The book is written to go through with ease and yet includes the essential details since it is crucial for the students and medical professionals to understand and be familiar with nuclear medicine since it is now an important component of modern medicine which should be utilized more effectively.

Abdelhamid H. Elgazzar, MD., FCAP

Acknowledgment

My thanks and gratitude goes to all who supported and helped to make this work a reality, particularly, Prof. Henry Wagner for his kind introduction for the book, Prof. Magda Elmonayeri for her sincere support, meticulous review, and sharp and valuable advices, Prof. Abdullatif Al-Bader for his comprehensive review and valuable advice and encouragement, and Mrs. Reham Haji, Mr. Ayman Taha, Dr. Eman Alenizi, Dr. Jarah Al-Tubaikh, Dr. Ahmed Gamal Afifi, Dr. Abdelmonem Omar, Mrs. Heba Issam, Miss Hanadi Al-Shammari, Mrs. Azza Al-Bunni, Mr. Mohamed Issa and Miss Aseel Alkandari for their help through the preparation.

Contents

Basic Considerations

1

Contents

1.1
Nuclear Medicine and Molecular Imaging

Nuclear medicine is a relatively new and rapidly changing specialty that depends on the evaluation of function. It is based on examining the regional chemistry of the living human body using radioactivity. Nuclear medicine simply is the medical use of radioactive agents to diagnose and treat patients.

Contrary to morphologic or structural modalities of diagnostic radiology such as x-ray computed tomography (CT) scan, nuclear medicine imaging is functional in nature since it depends on functional changes of the disease. It evaluates physiologic changes, metabolism, and more recently molecular alterations. Functional nuclear medicine studies including positron emission tomography (PET) provide useful information that cannot be obtained by morphologic modalities (Fig. 1.1).

A.H. Elgazzar, *A Concise Guide to Nuclear Medicine*,
DOI: 10.1007/978-3-642-19426-9_1, © Springer-Verlag Berlin Heidelberg 2011

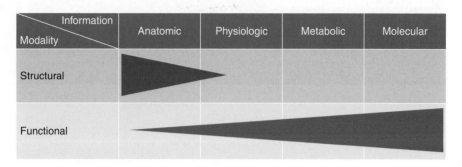

Fig. 1.1 Information provided by two main types of imaging modalities

Diagnostically it complements rather than competes with other imaging modalities (CT, MR, US) that depend predominantly on the morphology as it provides different information. The specialty has expanded and changed toward molecular imaging and therapy.

Anatomical abnormality is best diagnosed by morphologic modality's high-resolution examinations. Nuclear medicine studies are optimally utilized when the information sought is primarily physiological and biochemical in nature. These studies have advantages since they:

1. Are noninvasive and contain minimal risk for the patient
2. Have the ability to continuous monitoring over periods of time from several minutes to several hours without excessive radiation dose
3. Provide quantitation when imaging instruments are interfaced to computers
4. Can provide earlier diagnosis since physiological changes usually occur prior to morphological changes

1.2
Historical Background

The road to the current status of development of nuclear medicine imaging goes back to the discovery of x-rays by Roentgen (Fig. 1.2) in the year 1895 which is considered a start of discoveries in the field of ionizing radiation that opened the way for modern applications of radiation in the many fields including medicine.

Radioactivity, the basis of physiologic imaging, was discovered in 1896 by Becquerel (Fig. 1.3) which was further refined and defined by Anthony and Marie Curie (Figs. 1.4 and 1.5).

This was followed by several developments of morphologic imaging. Ultrasonography (US) was found in the 1950s while CT was in 1970s and MRI in the eighties. Radioactivity has been used in medicine by detecting activity by counting probes and later by imaging scanners and then cameras. Gamma camera was found in 1950s which was developed progressively later on with tomographic capability and multihead detectors (Figs. 1.6–1.8). More recently, Positron emission tomography (PET) signaled the main birth of molecular imaging which was further strengthened by merging morphologic and functional modalities (Fig. 1.9). Functional capability of US along with nanotechnology-based and optical imaging have added to the scope of molecular imaging technology.

Fig. 1.2 Roentgen

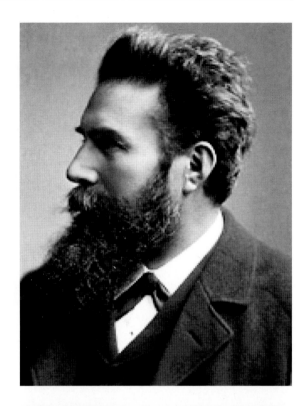

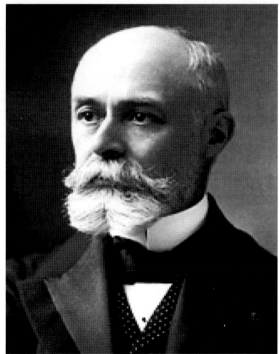

Fig. 1.3 Becquerel

Fig. 1.4 Pierre Curie

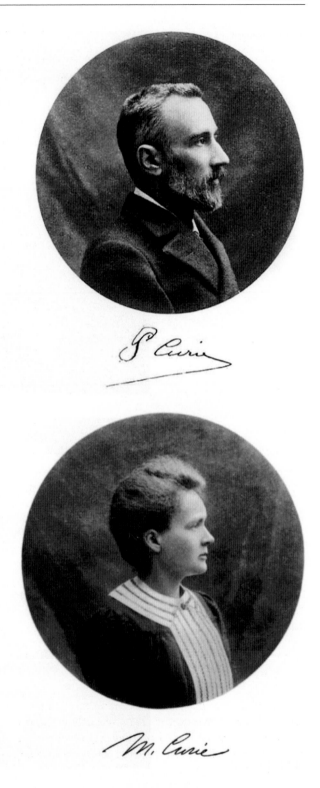

Fig. 1.5 Marie Curie

Fig. 1.6 Gamma camera with a single head

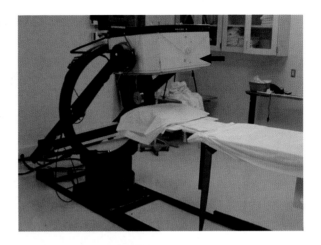

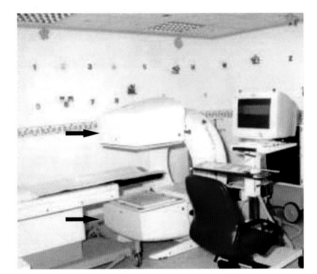

Fig. 1.7 Dual-headed gamma camera

1.3
Scientific Basis of Nuclear Medicine

1.3.1
Atomic Structure

Atoms initially were thought of as no more than small pieces of matter. Our understanding that they have an inner structure has its root in the observations of earlier physicists that the atoms of which matter is composed contain electrons of negative charge. While the atom as a whole is electrically neutral, it seemed obvious that it must also contain something with a

Fig. 1.8 Triple-headed
gamma camera. Note the
three detectors (*arrow
heads*)

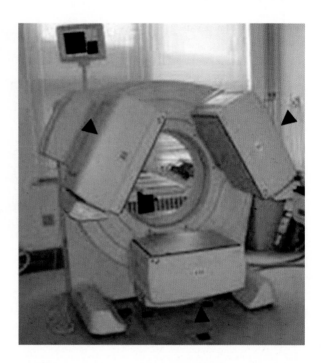

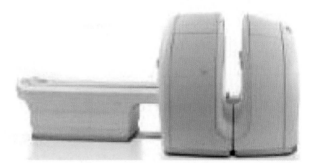

Fig. 1.9 PET/CT

positive charge to balance the negative charge of the electrons. Then it was confirmed that
the atom has negatively charged electrons orbiting a central group of particles forming the
positively charged nucleus (Fig. 1.10). Like the atom itself, the atomic nucleus also has an
inner structure (Fig. 1.10) that can be described as a tightly bound cluster of protons and
neutrons. The nucleus consists of two types of particles: protons, which carry a positive
charge, and neutrons, which carry no charge. The general term for protons and neutrons is
nucleons. The nucleons have a much greater mass than electrons. Protons naturally repel
each other since they are positively charged; however, there is a powerful binding force
called the nuclear force that holds the nucleons together very tightly. Nuclear binding force
is strong enough to overcome the electrical repulsion between the positively charged protons.

Fig. 1.10 Diagram of an atom

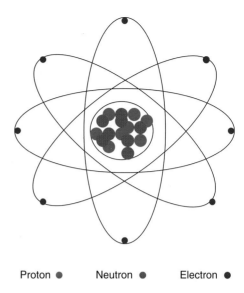

Proton ●   Neutron ●   Electron ●

The energy required to overcome the nuclear force is called the nuclear binding energy. Typical binding energies are in the range of 6–9 million electron volts (MeV) (approximately one thousand to one million times the electron binding force).

1.3.2
Isotopes

Each atom of any sample of an element has the same number of protons (the same Z: atomic number) in its nucleus. Lead found anywhere in the world will always be composed of atoms with 82 protons. The same does not apply, however, to the number of neutrons in the nucleus. An isotope of an element is a particular variation of the nuclear composition of the atoms of that element. The number of protons (Z: atomic number) is unchanged, but the number of neutrons (N) varies. Since the number of neutrons changes, the total number of neutrons and protons (A: the atomic mass) changes.

1.3.3
Radioactivity

A nucleus not in its stable state will adjust itself until it is stable either by ejecting portions of its nucleus or by emitting energy in the form of photons (gamma rays). This process is referred to as radioactive decay.

The unstable isotopes lie above or below the Nuclear Stability Curve. These unstable isotopes attempt to reach the stability curve by splitting into fragments, in a process called Fission, or by emitting particles and/or energy in the form of radiation. This latter process is called Radioactivity. The term radioactivity refers to the spontaneous emission of charged particles or photons by an atomic nucleus that is in an unstable status. This event is called a nuclear transformation, decay, or disintegration. Each decay event involves loss of mass or charge. Unstable isotopes, for instance, those that have too many protons to remain a stable entity are called radioactive isotopes and referred to as radioisotopes for short. The term radionuclide is also sometimes used. When this material is coupled with a chemical to carry it to a specific organ (carrier) it is referred to as radiopharmaceutical.

1.3.4
Radiopharmaceuticals

One of the major contributions of nuclear medicine is the development of radiopharmaceuticals. These are drugs that have been synthesized with radioactive components, which allow the drugs to be followed within the human body. Radioactivity also permits researchers to determine how much of the drug remains in the liver and in other organs, and how much is excreted by the kidneys. Since the physiological approach defines a disease in terms of the failure of a normal physiological or biochemical process, the nuclear medicine diagnostic procedures involve four types of physiologic measurement: (a) regional blood flow, transport, and cellular localization of various molecules; (b) metabolism and bioenergetics of tissues; (c) physiological function of organs; and (d) intracellular and intercellular communication.

A number of radiopharmaceuticals have been designed and developed over the past four decades to image the function of many organs and tissue.

The uptake and retention of radiopharmaceuticals by different tissues and organs involve many different mechanisms such as simple diffusion, active transport, facilitated diffusion, phagocytosis, metabolic trapping, cell proliferation, cell sequestration, and cell migration (Table 1.1).

Table 1.1 Common radiopharmaceuticals used in medicine

Radiopharmaceutical	Common clinical use (s)	Mechanism
Tc99m pertechnetate	Thyroid gland imaging	Trapping
Tc99m methylene diphosphonate (Tc99m MDP)	Bone imaging	Adsorption by hydroxyapatite crystals
Tc99m iminodiacetic acid (IDA) derivatives	Hepatobiliary imaging	Active uptake by hepatocytes and excretion with bile
Tc99m macroaggregated albumin particles (Tc99m MAA)	Lung perfusion imaging	Blockage of capillaries and precapillary arterioles
Tc99m MAG-3	Renal dynamic imaging	Tubular excretion
Gallium-67 citrate	Tumor and infection imaging	Iron containing globulins binding
Labeled white blood cells	Infection imaging	Cell migration
Flourine-18 fluorodeoxyglucose (F-18-FDG)	Tumor imaging	Active transport to cells (glucose analogue)

1.4
Technical Principles of Nuclear Medicine

A radiopharmaceutical is administered to the patient and it accumulates in the organ of inter-est. Gamma-rays are emitted in all directions from the organ and those heading in the direction of the gamma camera enter the crystal and produce scintillations. A flash of light appears on the screen of the Cathode ray oscilloscope (CRO) at a point related to where the scintillation occurred within the NaI (Tl) crystal. An image of the distribution of the radiopharmaceutical within the organ is therefore formed. The form of imaging, Planar imaging (Fig. 1.11a) pro-duces a two-dimensional image of a three-dimensional object. As a result images contain no depth information and some details can be superimposed on top of each other and obscured or partially obscured as a result. This is also a feature of conventional x-ray imaging.

Tomographic images are also obtained using gamma cameras or positron emission tomographic cameras where images are recorded at a series of angles around the patient. These images are then subjected to a form of digital image processing in order to compute images of slices through the patient (Fig. 1.11b).

New procedures combine PET or gamma camera with computed x-ray tomography (CT) scans and more recently with Magnetic Resonance Imaging (MRI) to give fusion of the two images (PET/CT, PET/MR and SPECT/CT), and enables better diagnosis than with tradi-tional gamma camera or PET alone. It is a very powerful and significant tool which pro-vides information that cannot be obtained from any of these modalities alone on a wide variety of benign and malignant diseases.

1.5
Scope of Nuclear Medicine

Although nuclear medicine imaging is still widely underappreciated and underused by the medical communities, it continues to provide advances for diagnosis and treatment of many diseases, as well as many fundamental insights into the complex workings of the human body. The vast majority of the specialty is diagnostic while the smaller portion is therapeutic which is expanding quickly.

1.5.1
Diagnostic Nuclear Medicine

Over 10,000 hospitals worldwide use radioisotopes in medicine, and 85–90% of the procedures are for diagnosis. The most common radioisotope used in diagnosis is technetium-99, with more than 30 million procedures per year worldwide.

Among developed countries, in the USA there are some 18 million nuclear medicine procedures per year among 305 million people, and in Europe about 10 million among 500 million people. In Australia there are about 560,000 per year among 21 million people.

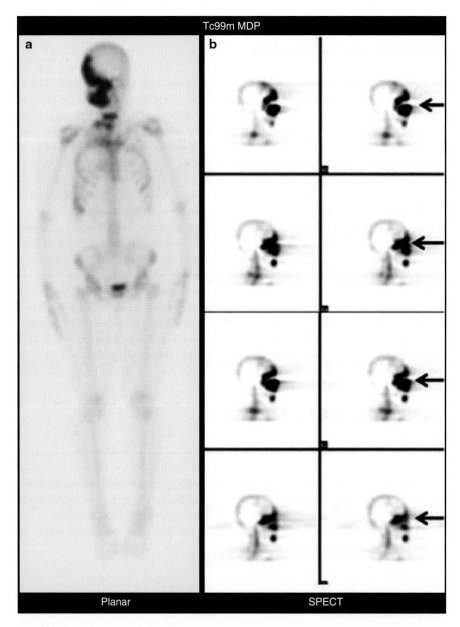

Fig. 1.11 (**a**) Two dimension (*planar image*) bone image showing abnormality in the right face (Fibrous dysplasia). (**b**) Tomographic images of the skull of the same patient showing slices of the skull and more details of the abnormality (*arrows*)

Nuclear medicine is used to diagnose many diseases of many organs using unstable agents that emit gamma rays from within the body as they decay. These tracers are generally short-lived isotopes linked to chemical compounds which carry the molecules to desired location which permit specific physiological processes to be scrutinized. They can be given by injection, inhalation, or orally. The photons emitted are detected by a camera which can view organs from many different angles. The camera builds up an image from the points from which radiation is emitted; this image is enhanced by a computer and viewed by a physician on a monitor for indications of abnormal conditions (Fig. 1.12).

This specialty illustrates a team model in medical practice since physicians, technologists, radiopharmacists, physicists, radiation safety officer, and computer engineer are needed to practice. For interpretation of images, physicians need the patient's medical history, laboratory and radiologic procedures previously done, previous nuclear studies, and perform physical examination when needed.

1.5.2
Nuclear Medicine Therapy

Nuclear medicine offers treatment options for several diseases and this component is expanding rapidly. Examples of the therapeutic applications include thyroid hyperactivity, bone pain due to metastases, certain joint diseases, blood diseases, and tumors as thyroid cancer and lymphomas. The treatment using radionuclides usually consists of a single administration with very few side effects.

Rapidly dividing cells are particularly sensitive to damage by radiation. For this reason, some cancerous growths can be controlled or eliminated by irradiating the area containing the growth. External irradiation (sometimes called teletherapy) can be carried out using a gamma beam from a radioactive cobalt-60 source, but the much more versatile linear accelerators are now being utilized as a high-energy x-ray source.

Internal radionuclide therapy is by administering or planting a small radiation source, usually a gamma or beta emitter, in the target area. Short-range radiotherapy is known as brachytherapy, and this is becoming the main means of treatment. Iodine-131 is commonly used to treat thyroid cancer, probably the most successful kind of cancer treatment. It is also used to treat nonmalignant thyroid disorders.

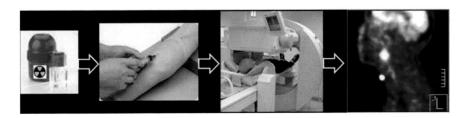

Fig. 1.12 Illustration of the technique of nuclear medicine imaging

1.6
Summary

The field of nuclear medicine is an interdisciplinary approach since it interacts with multiple medical specialists. Nuclear medicine has developed in the past 50 years and is now a fully established medical specialty. It depends on the use of unsealed radionuclides and the tracer principle. Nuclear medicine combines medicine and basic biological sciences which originally had their roots in the fields of radiology, internal medicine, and pathology. Although nuclear medicine is primarily a clinical diagnostic discipline, it uses physical-chemical principles and requires a background in such areas as physiology, biochemistry, mathematics, physics, chemistry, computer sciences, and statistics.

A wide selection of radiopharmaceuticals is available for single-photon imaging designed to study numerous physiologic processes within the body. Static, dynamic, gated, and tomographic modes of single-photon acquisition can be performed. Dual-photon imaging is the principle underlying positron emission tomography (PET) and is fundamentally tomographic. PET has expanded rapidly due to the clinical impact of the radiopharmaceutical ^{18}F-fluorodeoxyglucose, a glucose analogue used for imaging of malignancy. The fusion of nuclear medicine tomographic images with anatomic CT is evolving into a dominant imaging technique.

Nuclear medicine diagnostic procedures yield mainly functional information and contribute to the management of a wide spectrum of diseases. Therapeutic nuclear medicine utilizes targeted radiation damage at the disease site and has applications in both benign and malignant diseases. The future directions for nuclear medicine include increasing use of tomographic methods and the development of radiopharmaceuticals which localize on receptors.

Further Reading

Cember H (2009) Introduction to health physics. McGraw-Hill, New York
Cuocolo A, Breatnach E (2010) Multimodality imaging in Europe: a survey by the European Association of Nuclear Medicine (EANM) and the European Society of Radiology (ESR). Eur J Nucl Med Mol Imaging 37:163–167
Ernest Lawrence http://en.wikipedia.org/wiki/Ernest_Lawrence
Ernest Rutherford http://en.wikipedia.org/wiki/Ernest_Rutherford
Henkin RE (2006) Nuclear medicine, 2nd edn. Mosby, St. Louis
Henri Becquerel http://en.wikipedia.org/wiki/Henri_Becquerel
James Chadwick http://en.wikipedia.org/wiki/James_Chadwick
JJ Thomson http://www.aip.org/history/electron/jjthomson.htm
Lide D (2001) CRC handbook of chemistry and physics. Boca Raton, London/New York
Marie Curie http://en.wikipedia.org/wiki/Marie_Curie
Saha G (2001) Physics and radiobiology of nuclear medicine, 2nd edn. Springer, Berlin
Wagner HN Jr (2006) A personal history of nuclear medicine. Springer, New York

Genitourinary System

2

Contents

2.1
Introduction

Scintigraphy has provided a unique tool for the noninvasive evaluation of renal pathophysiology, and there is still a rapid increase in the scope and number of radionuclide renal studies. This chapter familiarizes the reader with the most frequently used procedures encountered in nuclear medicine in genitourinary system. These include studies for renovascular hypertension, urinary tract obstruction, urinary tract infection, renal transplant complications, and testicular torsion.

A.H. Elgazzar, *A Concise Guide to Nuclear Medicine*,
DOI: 10.1007/978-3-642-19426-9_2, © Springer-Verlag Berlin Heidelberg 2011

2.2
Radiopharmaceuticals

Several radiotracers are used for imaging genitourinary system conditions. These include renal radiopharmaceuticals for dynamic and static studies, Tc99m sulfur calloid for direct Vesico-ureteral reflux study and Tc99m-pertechnetate for scrotal imaging.

Renal radiopharmaceuticals can be described in two broad classes – those that are excreted rapidly into the urine and those that are retained for prolonged periods in the renal parenchyma.

1. Rapidly excreted radiopharmaceuticals are used in dynamic imaging studies to assess individual renal function and include the following:
   (a) ^{99m}Tc-mercaptoacetyltriglycine (MAG3) which is the agent of choice, is 90% protein bound, and excreted almost exclusively by the renal tubules. High renal-to-background count ratios provide excellent images and permit visualization of poorly functioning kidneys.
   (b) ^{99m}Tc-diethylenetriamine penta-acetic acid (DTPA) which was the most popular radiopharmaceutical in its category prior to the introduction of ^{99m}Tc-MAG3. It shows little protein binding (about 5%) and is excreted exclusively by glomerular filtration. Renal uptake of ^{99m}Tc-DTPA is limited because only 20% of the renal blood flow is filtered by the glomeruli. The 20% extraction fraction is considerably lower than that of ^{99m}Tc-MAG3 and yields lower renal-to-background uptake ratios. However it is less costly and may be used as an alternative to ^{99m}Tc-MAG3, particularly if a quantitative estimate of GFR is also needed.
2. The slowly excreted radiopharmaceuticals include ^{99m}Tc-dimercaptosuccinic acid (DMSA) and ^{99m}Tc-glucoheptonate. Prolonged cortical retention of these radiopharmaceuticals allows the assessment of parenchymal morphology, and since accumulation occurs only in functioning tubules, uptake can be quantified to assess accurately the differential renal function. The preferred agent, Technetium-99 m-DMSA, is 90% protein bound and accumulates in functioning tubules. Since very little of the radiotracer is excreted, interference from collecting system activity, particularly on delayed images, is minimal. A total of about 40% of the administered amount is accumulated in the renal cortex.

2.3
Imaging Studies

(a) Renal scintigraphy

According to the types of renal radiopharmaceuticals, renal scintigraphy can be of dynamic or static nature.

– Dynamic studies are obtained using the rapidly excreted radiopharmaceuticals. Dynamic studies start by rapid acquisition of image frames upon injection of the

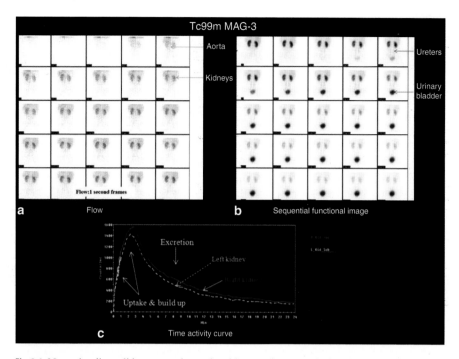

Fig. 2.1 Normal radionuclide renography study with normal symmetrical perfusion as seen on flow phase (**a**), function as noted on sequential functioning images presented as 1 min frames (**b**) and time–activity curves (**c**)

tracer to follow activity while passing through the blood vessels till reaching the kidneys to evaluate the blood flow (Fig. 2.1a). This phase is followed by another series of imaging frames every 10–20 s of the kidney to evaluate the kidney functional handling of the radiotracer (Fig. 2.1b). This phase will then be computer processed to generate time–activity curve (renogram) for both kidneys to illustrate the uptake, build up, and excretion of the radiopharmaceutical by each kidney (Fig. 2.1c) and generate the percent contribution of each kidney to the total renal function (split or differential renal function).

- Static studies using slowly secreted radiopharmaceuticals, particularly Tc99m DMSA, are acquired 3 h after intravenous injection of the radiotracer and optionally up to 24 h based on the individual case and the kidney function. Anterior, posterior, left, and right posterior oblique views are obtained. These studies are predominantly used to accurately determine the split renal function and in cases of urinary tract infections to evaluate the changes including cortical scars: Using the anterior and posterior views the split renal function is calculated by the geometric mean of the background subtracted kidney counts.

(b) Vesicoureteral reflux study

(c) Scrotal imaging study

2.4
Clinical Uses

2.4.1
Dynamic Renal Scintigraphy

- Evaluation of renal perfusion and function
- Diagnosis of renovascular hypertension
- Diagnosis and follow-up of urinary tract obstruction
- Evaluation of renal transplant complications

2.4.2
Static Renal Scintigraphy

- Urinary tract infections
- Evaluation of renal masses
- Quantitating differential renal function
- Congenital renal malformations (horseshoe kidney)

2.4.3
Vesicoureteral Reflux Study

Diagnosis and follow-up of vesicoureteral reflux

2.4.4
Scrotal Imaging

Diagnosis of testicular torsion and inflammation

2.5
Commonly Used Applications

2.5.1
Diagnosis of Renovascular Hypertension

The role of the renin-angiotensin system, i.e., maintenance of systemic blood pressure, is well played in such conditions as hypotension and shock. In significant renal artery stenosis, however, activation of the renin-angiotensin system is a mixed blessing, limiting a fall in GFR but causing systemic (renovascular) hypertension. Systemic blood pressure is maintained primarily by increase in vascular tone and retention of sodium and water, while a sharp reduction in GFR is prevented by increase in the glomerular capillary hydrostatic pressure.

Glomerular capillary hydrostatic pressure is modulated by the tone of the afferent and efferent glomerular arterioles. Increased tone in the efferent arteriole or decreased tone (increased flow) in the afferent arteriole raises capillary hydrostatic pressure and GFR, while decreased tone in the efferent arteriole or increased tone (decreased flow) in the afferent arteriole lowers GFR.

The scintigraphic diagnosis of renovascular hypertension is based on the demonstration of changes in renal physiology following the administration of an ACE inhibitor. Angiotensin II, formed by the activation of the renin-angiotensin system, helps maintain GFR by increasing the tone of the efferent glomerular arteriole which, in turn, raises the glomerular capillary hydrostatic pressure. These changes are reversed by ACE inhibitors, which block the conversion of angiotensin I to angiotensin II. Consequently, there is a sharp drop in GFR and in proximal tubular urine flow.

Decreased GFR and tubular flow after the administration of an ACE inhibitor will result in decreased uptake and prolonged cortical retention of ^{99m}Tc-DTPA, which is excreted by glomerular filtration. On the other hand, ^{99m}Tc-MAG3, which is a tubular and blood flow agent, shows only prolonged cortical retention without apparent decreased uptake since renal blood flow generally is not significantly changed (Figs. 2.2 and 2.3). Rarely, uptake of ^{99m}Tc-MAG3 may actually decrease, presumably due to a fall in blood pressure below a critical level required to maintain perfusion in the stenotic kidney.

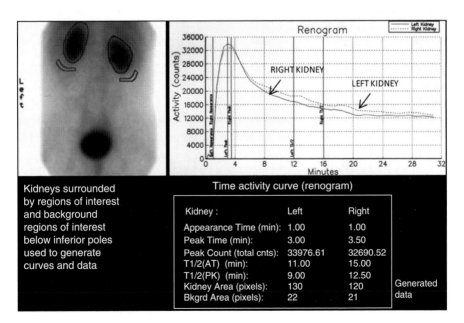

Kidney :	Left	Right
Appearance Time (min):	1.00	1.00
Peak Time (min):	3.00	3.50
Peak Count (total cnts):	33976.61	32690.52
T1/2(AT) (min):	11.00	15.00
T1/2(PK) (min):	9.00	12.50
Kidney Area (pixels):	130	120
Bkgrd Area (pixels):	22	21

Kidneys surrounded by regions of interest and background regions of interest below inferior poles used to generate curves and data

Time activity curve (renogram)

Generated data

Fig. 2.2 Normal captopril study with normal excretion and no cortical retention of activity bilaterally (*arrows*)

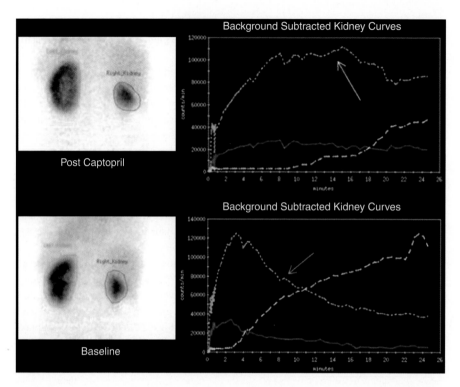

Fig. 2.3 Abnormal captopril study showing retention of activity in right kidney with Captopril on time–activity curve (*arrow*) compared to the baseline study (*lower curve*) where there is good clearance (*arrow*)

2.5.2
Urinary Tract Obstruction

The most commonly used radiotracer for diuretic renography is Tc99m mercaptoacetyl-triglycine (MAG-3).

Urinary tract obstruction may be high grade complete or partial, and it may occur at various locations including the ureteropelvic junction (UPJ), ureterovesical junction (UVJ), and bladder outlet. The clinical consequences are quite dramatic and predictable in an acute and complete obstruction, but not in a partial and chronic one, exemplified by UPJ obstruction in children. Chronic UPJ obstruction may eventually lead to renal cortical atrophy.

Diuretic renography is based on the premise that increased urine flow resulting after furosemide administration causes rapid "washout" of radiotracer from the unobstructed collecting system (Fig. 2.4), but delayed washout if obstruction is present (Figs. 2.5 and 2.6). The washout half-time following diuretic injection is determined from the time-activity curve. A half time of 10 min or less is considered normal, 10–20 min equivocal, and more

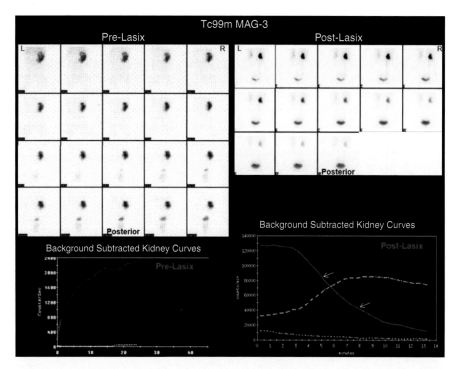

Fig. 2.4 A radionuclide diuretic renography study illustrating hold up of activity in the right functioning kidney by the end of pre-lasix study with rapid washout on post-lasix study which is clearly illustrated on the time–activity curve. These exemplify the nonobstructed pattern

than 20 min abnormal. Given the dynamic nature of UPJ obstruction, however, a number of factors may influence the diuretic renogram and must be taken into consideration for a proper assessment.

2.5.3
Urinary Tract Infection

Pyelonephritis refers to infection of the renal tubules, pelvis, and interstitium, and it has a wide spectrum of clinical presentations. While the clinical diagnosis is obvious when characteristic manifestations of flank or back pain, fever, and bacteriuria are present, pyelonephritis may be missed if symptoms are absent or referable only to the lower urinary tract. Acute pyelonephritis requires more vigorous treatment than lower urinary tract infection, and, left untreated, it can lead to scarring and renal insufficiency. Consequently, identification of renal involvement is critical in children with suspected urinary tract infection, and parenchymal scintigraphy with the tubular agent, Tc-99 m-dimercaptosuccinic acid (DMSA) can play an important role in their diagnostic evaluation.

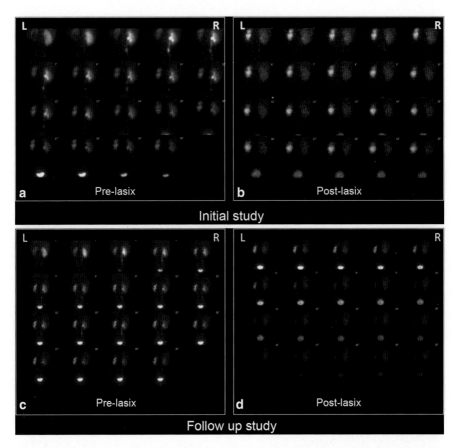

Fig. 2.5 Left-sided urine outflow obstruction in a 4-year-old patient with left hydronephrosis before (**a**) and after lasix injection (**b**). The preoperative study shows decreased uptake in the left kidney and slow accumulation of the radiotracer. After lasix injection there is retained activity in the left kidney due to poor response compared to right kidney which shows good uptake and complete clearance. The study was repeated after surgery and there is better uptake and accumulation of activity before lasix injection (**c**) and clearance of activity from the left kidney after lasix injection (**d**)

Ascending infection from the lower urinary tract is the usual mechanism for pyelonephritis. The infection appears to originate in the urethra or the vaginal introitus, which are colonized by enteric flora, predominantly *Escherichia coli*, and it is more common in females, presumably due to their shorter urethra. Structural abnormalities of the urinary tract such as vesicoureteral reflux and bladder outlet obstruction (which exacerbate reflux) are important predisposing factors, though often not demonstrable. Another predisposing factor appears to be an inborn increase in uroepithelial cell susceptibility to bacterial adherence, which facilitates bacterial ascent to the upper urinary tract. Finally, catheterization and sexual intercourse can allow urethral bacteria to enter the bladder. Ascending infection eventually reaches the renal calyces, from which microorganisms enter the parenchyma through the papillae by intrarenal reflux.

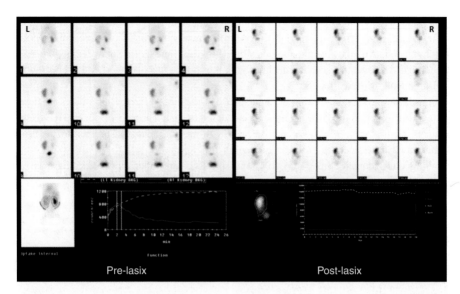

Fig. 2.6 A diuretic renography study in an adult patient illustrating obstructive pattern in the *left* side. Note the left kidney time–activity curve which shows no clearance before lasix (*arrow*) and no response to lasix (*arrow head*)

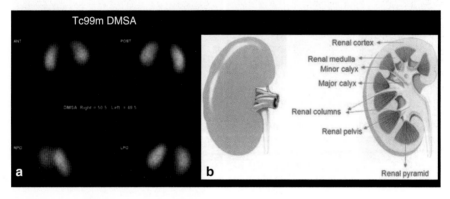

Fig. 2.7 Normal DMSA study with no cortical defects (**a**) and a diagram of normal kidney illustrating smooth surface and regular cortex (**b**)

Scarring of the renal parenchyma may result from pyelonephritis. It is a common cause of hypertension and, if sufficiently extensive, it can lead to progressive renal insufficiency and end-stage renal disease. Although vesicoureteral reflux is frequently associated with scarring, it is not a prerequisite for this condition.

Imaging of the renal parenchyma with ^{99m}Tc-DMSA offers a simple and accurate method for detecting acute pyelonephritis in the child with urinary tract infection. ^{99m}Tc-DMSA localizes in functioning proximal tubular cells and is not excreted in significant amounts, so that imaging at 4–24 h after radiopharmaceutical administration reveals primarily cortical uptake without interfering activity in the collecting system (Fig. 2.7).

A cortical defect due to pyelonephritis is characterized by preservation of renal contour, whereas scarring (from a previous infection) typically results in volume contraction, although the two may be indistinguishable (Figs. 2.8 and 2.9). Such distinction may become less relevant as scarring declines with the routine use of ^{99m}Tc-DMSA imaging in children with urinary infection.

In addition to imaging during the acute phase of the disease, follow-up studies are done to confirm resolution of the pyelonephritic defect(s) and absence of cortical scarring. Patients with scars are followed periodically with imaging and measurement of relative function for assessment of progressive renal insufficiency.

Magnetic resonance imaging (MRI) and spiral CT are other modalities that may be helpful in the evaluation of pyelonephritis.

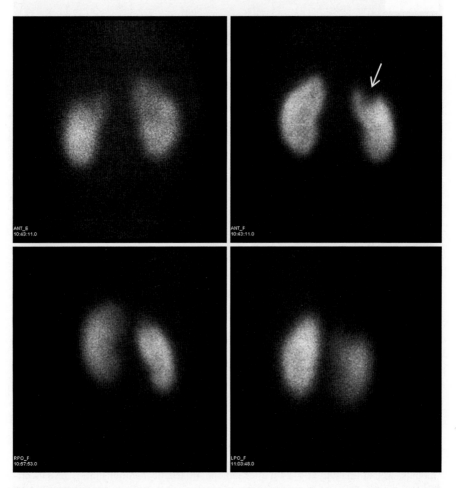

Fig. 2.8 Tc99m DMSA study of a 4-year-old female child with UTI. Study shows defect in the right upper pole (*arrow*)

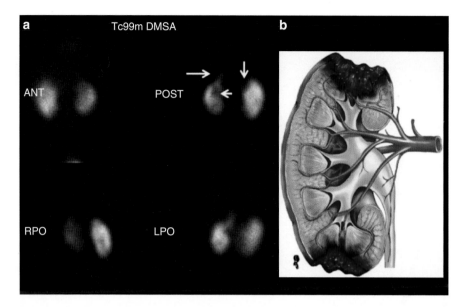

Fig. 2.9 (**a**) Tc99m DMSA study demonstrating bilateral upper pole defects and a midleft kidney defect (*arrows*). (**b**) Illustrates how scars affect the kidney contour compared with the normal contour as seen in Fig. 2.7b

2.5.4
Vesicoureteral Reflux

Urinary tract infection is a common problem in children. Approximately 40% of patients with upper urinary tract infection have vesicoureteral reflux. Misdiagnosed or inadequately treated urinary tract infection can lead to serious complications such as hypertension and chronic renal failure.

Direct radionuclide cystography using Tc99m Sulfur calloid is a method to evaluate for vesicoureteral reflux, which has several advantages including significantly less gonadal radiation when compared with conventional radiographic technique, voiding cystourethrogram (VCUG). The international radiologic grading includes 5 grades using some detailed anatomy such as characterization of the fornices that is impossible to achieve by scintigraphic studies. Accordingly a more simplified scintigraphic grading attempt classifies reflux into 3 grades (Table 2.1 and Fig. 2.10) Mild (I), Moderate (II) and Severe (III).

The test is recognized for the initial evaluation of females with urinary tract infection for reflux, diagnosis of familial reflux, and for the evaluation of vesicoureteral reflux after medical and/or surgical management (Fig. 2.11).

Table 2.1 Scintigraphic grading for vesicoureteral reflux

Mild (Grade I)	Reflux into ureter
Moderate (Grade II)	Reflux into pelvocalyceal system
Severe (Grade III)	Reflux into pelvocalyceal system with dilated pelvis or both pelvis and ureter

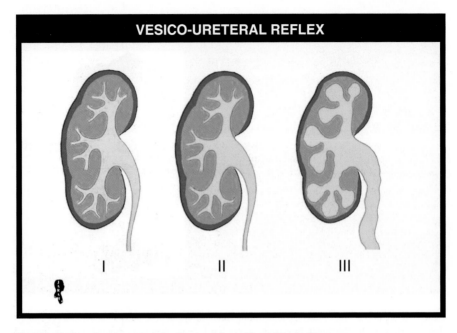

Fig. 2.10 Grades of vesico-ureteral reflux used for radionuclide studies

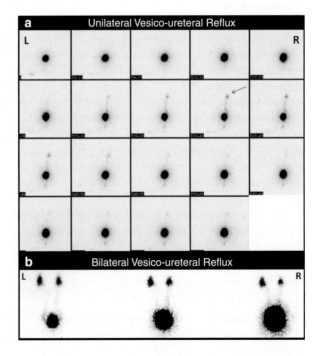

Fig. 2.11 (**a**) Vesicoureteral reflux study showing right side grade II reflux (*arrow*). (**b**) Bilateral vesicoureteral grade III reflux

2.5.5
Evaluation of Renal Transplant Complications

Advances in our understanding of the pathophysiology of renal transplants over the past several years have resulted in significant improvement in renal graft survival and an increase in the number of transplantations. The key factors influencing survival are donor–recipient histocompatibility and donor status (living related, living unrelated, or cadaver). Graft survival is best when the donor is an HLA-identical sibling, and better for living-related than for cadaver donors with similar HLA matches. A host of other factors, including harvesting and transplantation technique, cold ischemia time (between harvest and transplantation), donor/recipient age, recurrence of primary renal disease, and race also play an important role in graft survival. Renal scintigraphy helps evaluate the perfusion and function of transplanted kidney (Fig. 2.12) and detect and follow

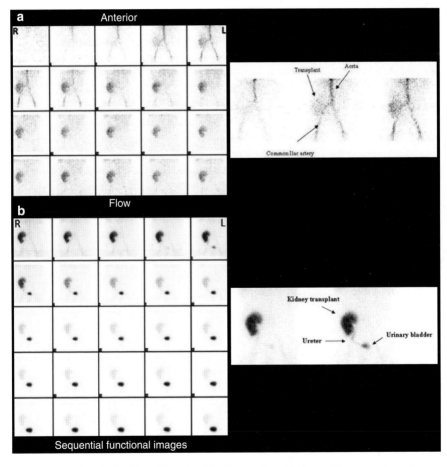

Fig. 2.12 Normal perfusion (**a**) and function (**b**) of a transplanted kidney with representative images with labeled diagrams illustrating the structures on images

postoperative complications. The surgical and medical complications of renal transplantation are considered below.

2.5.5.1
Surgical Complications

Scintigraphic studies can be used effectively to evaluate urine extravasation (Fig. 2.13), ureteral obstruction, hematoma, lymphocele, and renal artery stenosis

2.5.5.2
Medical Complications

Acute Tubular Necrosis

Acute tubular necrosis (ATN), characterized by ischemic necrosis of the tubular epithelial cells and decreased GFR, is frequently associated with cadaver renal transplants. Possible causes are hypotension/hypovolemia in the donor and prolonged interval between harvest and transplantation. After transplantation, urine output usually starts to decrease within the first 24 h or so and improves spontaneously after a few days, although ATN may occasionally last a few weeks. It is often difficult to make a clinical distinction between ATN and rejection in the post-transplantation period. A clear scintigraphic distinction between these two conditions also has remained elusive, for two reasons. First, the scintigraphic diagnosis of ATN rests on the premise that graft perfusion is preserved despite decreasing function, in contrast to rejection, where both perfusion and function decrease. However, depending on the severity/stage of ATN, graft perfusion may vary. Second, ATN and acute rejection may coexist.

Recovery of the condition can best be ascertained by serial scintigraphy.

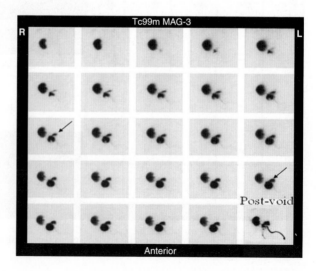

Fig. 2.13 Tc 99 m MAG-3 study obtained for a patient after renal transplantation. There is extravasation of activity indicating postoperative leak (*arrow*)

Rejection

According to Banff Classification rejection can be of the following types:

1. Antibody-mediated rejection: Two types of antibody-mediated rejection are described, immediate or hyperacute, and delayed or accelerated acute. Hyperacute rejection is caused by preformed antidonor antibodies. Rejection may begin within minutes or hours and is usually apparent during surgery. Scintigraphy shows a photopenic region corresponding to the avascular graft. Fortunately, hyperacute rejection is rare and largely preventable by appropriate screening tests.

   Accelerated acute rejection may be considered a "slow" variant of hyperacute rejection, mediated primarily by antidonor antibodies. It usually occurs on the second or third day following transplantation, after allograft function has been established. Scintigraphy generally shows poor radiotracer uptake in the graft.

2. Acute/active rejection: Acute rejection is the most frequent type of rejection confronting the nuclear medicine physician (Fig. 2.14). It is most common in the first 4 weeks following transplantation but may occur at any time between 3 days and 10 or more years.

3. Chronic/sclerosing allograft nephropathy: Chronic/sclerosing nephropathy generally occurs 6 months to years after transplantation. It may be related to a number of causes including chronic rejection, hypertension, an infectious/noninfectious inflammatory process, and effects of medications.

2.5.6
Diagnosis of Testicular Torsion

Testicular torsion is an emergency condition which needs immediate diagnosis and management. In most institutions, Doppler ultrasound is used most commonly as the

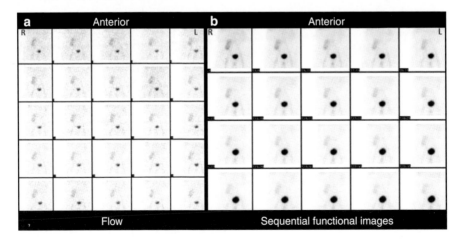

Fig. 2.14 Tc 99 m MAG-3 study for a patient with renal transplantation showing decreased perfusion (**a**) and function (**b**) of the graft illustrating the typical scintigraphic findings of rejection

standard imaging technique of choice to confirm the diagnosis in most cases. Scintigraphy is used when color Doppler is inadequate, raising doubts about the suspected torsion. Recent studies, however, comparing both modalities indicate that scintigraphy is more accurate for the diagnosis of testicular torsion. The study is performed using Tc99m-pertechnetate injected IV and show normally symmetrical and uniform perfusion (Fig. 2.15). In acute torsion, there is decreased perfusion to the affected side (Fig. 2.16) while in epididymitis which may be clinically difficult to differentiate from

Fig. 2.15 Normal scrotal imaging study obtained using Tc99m pertechnetate

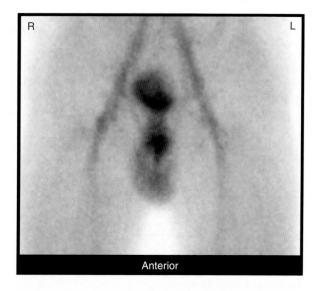

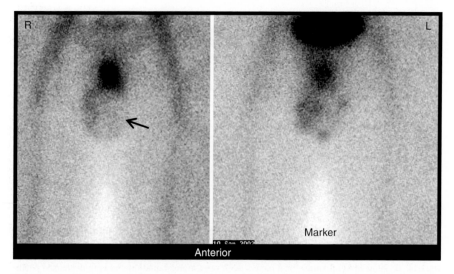

Fig. 2.16 Scrotal imaging study illustrating *left* side acute torsion indicated by decreased uptake (*arrow*)

torsion the study shows increased perfusion (Fig. 2.17). Torsion of long duration (missed torsion) appears as an area of decreased perfusion surrounded by a rim of increased uptake (Fig. 2.18).

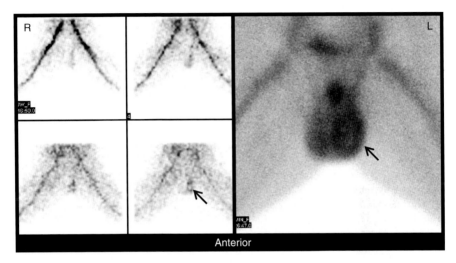

Fig. 2.17 Scrotal imaging study showing increased activity in the *left* side (*arrow*) in a case of epididymitis

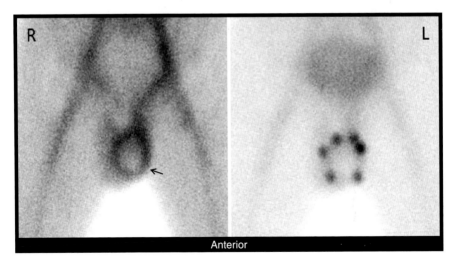

Fig. 2.18 Scrotal imaging study demonstrating the pattern of torsion of long duration in the *left* side (*arrow*) with markers around the affected testicle (*right side*)

2.6
Summary

Radionuclide imaging plays a very important role in genitourinary diseases. It is instrumental in the diagnosis and follow-ups of urine outflow obstruction in adults and more importantly in pediatric age group. It also plays an important role in detecting complications of urinary tract infection and is part of the management protocols. It also helps in the detection and more importantly follow-up of vesicoureteral reflux and evaluation of renal transplantation and its complications. It helps differentiate testicular torsion from epididymitis/epididymo-orchitis and other conditions.

Further Reading

Conway JJ (1989) The principles and technical aspects of diuresis renographDy. J Nucl Med Technol 17:208–214

Haufe SE, Riedmüller K, Haberkorn U (2006) Nuclear medicine procedures for the diagnosis of acute and chronic renal failure. Nephron Clin Pract 103:c77–c84

Majd M, Rushton HG (1992) Renal cortical scintigraphy in the diagnosis of acute pyelonephritis. Semin Nucl Med 22:98–111

Mandell GA, Eggli DF, Gilday DL, Heyman S, Leonard JC, Miller JH, Nadel HR, Piepsz A, Treves ST (2003) Procedure guideline for radionuclide cystography in children 3.0. Society of Nuclear Medicine, Reston, 6 p

Piepsz A, Ham HR (2006) Pediatric applications of renal nuclear medicine. Semin Nucl Med 36:16–35

Sarkar SD, Singhal PC (2006) Basis of renal scintigraphy. In: Elgazzar AH (ed) Pathophysiologic basis of nuclear medicine, 2nd edn. Springer, Berlin/New York

Wu H, Sun S, Kao A, Chuang F, Lin C, Lee C (2002) Comparison of radionuclide imaging and ultrasonography in the differentiation of acute testicular torsion and inflammatory testicular disease. Clin Nucl Med 27:490–493

Digestive and Hepatobiliary System

3

Contents

3.1
Introduction

Several scintigraphic imaging procedures are being used to diagnose and follow-up gastrointestinal and hepatobiliary conditions. These functional studies provide information that are complementary to those of the morphologic studies and may not be demonstrated by them. The following is a brief discussion of the most common procedures.

3.2
Clinical Uses

- Evaluation of esophageal transit time
- Evaluation of gastric emptying
- Localization of lower gastrointestinal bleeding
- Detection of Meckel's diverticulum
- Evaluation of inflammatory bowel disease
- Diagnosis of hepatic hemangioma
- Diagnosis of acute cholecystitis
- Diagnosis of common bile duct obstruction
- Evaluation of neonatal hyperbilirubinemia
- Evaluation of complications after hepatobiliary surgery
- Diagnosis and follow-up of *Helicobacter pylori* infection and malabsorption

3.3
Evaluation of Esophageal Transit Time

Radionuclide esophageal transit study is sensitive in detecting esophageal disorders and its involvement in certain systemic disorders. The patient should fast for 4–6 h. A dose of 250–500 µCi Tc-99m-Sulfur colloid in 10 mL of water is taken through a straw. It is preferable to do the imaging in the supine position to eliminate the effect of gravity; images of 1 s each are acquired to characterize the esophageal transit. Delayed images at 10 min may be helpful in patients with significant stasis of radioactivity in the esophagus.

A time–activity curve can be generated; the esophageal transit time is the time interval between the peak activity of the proximal esophageal curve and the peak activity of the distal esophageal curve. The normal transit time is 15 s, with a distinct peak in each third of the esophagus. Prolonged transit time might be found in several esophageal and systemic disorders (Table 3.1).

Table 3.1 Main causes of prolonged esophageal transit

1. Achalasia
2. Progressive systemic sclerosis
3. Diffuse esophageal spasm
4. Nutcracker esophagus
5. Zenker's diverticulum
6. Esophageal stricture
7. Esophageal tumors

3.4
Detection of Gastroesophageal Reflux

Gastroesophageal reflux is a condition characterized reduction of the lower esophageal sphincter resulting in leaking of the stomach acidity into the esophagus. Radionuclide study to detect and follow-up of the disease is particularly useful in pediatric age-group. The patient should fast for 4 h. The dose is 0.5–1 mCi Tc-99m-sulfur colloid in 300 mL of acidic orange juice or water (milk or formula in pediatric age group). Imaging is performed with the subject in a supine position at a rate of 1 frame/10 s for 60 min. Reflux is seen as distinct spikes of activity into the esophagus (Fig. 3.1). The episodes of reflux are graded as high or low level, by duration (less or more than 10 s), and by their relationship to meal ingestion.

This scintigraphic study has 89% correlation with the acid reflux test. Evidence of pulmonary aspiration is valuable in the pediatric age-group.

3.5
Evaluation of Gastric Emptying

The patient should fast overnight. The dose is 0.5–1.0 mCi Tc-99m-SC mixed with egg white or liver pâté as a solid meal. Dynamic images can be taken for 60 min and if necessary, static delayed images are taken every 15 min until at least 50% of the stomach activity (content) has gone into the bowel.

Normally, the stomach should empty 50% of the activity measured at time zero by 90 min. Solids leave the stomach in a linear fashion (Fig. 3.2). Gastric emptying may be acutely or chronically delayed or abnormally rapid (Tables 3.2–3.4).

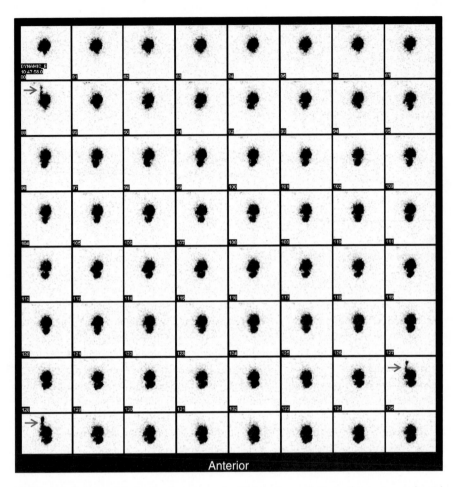

Fig. 3.1 Activity is noted in the esophagus in several frames (*arrows*) illustrating gastroesophageal reflux

3.6
Lower Gastrointestinal Bleeding Localization

Gastrointestinal bleeding (GIB) is divided into upper and lower. The upper gastrointestinal bleeding is defined as bleeding proximal to the ligament of Treitz while the lower bleeding is distal to the ligament. Radionuclide study is useful in the detection of the lower GI bleeding.

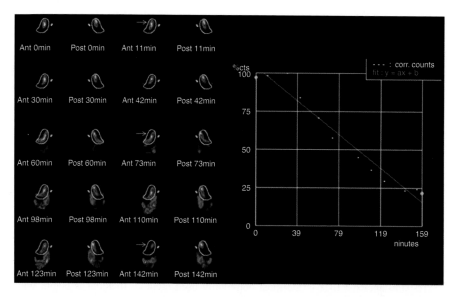

Fig. 3.2 An example of normal gastric emptying study with progressive decrease of activity in the stomach (*arrows*) over the study time which is also reflected on the slope of time-activity curve

Table 3.2 Common causes of acutely delayed gastric emptying

1. Stress (as in cold or pain)
2. Drugs (morphine, anticholinergics, levodopa, nicotine, beta blockers)
3. Hyperglycemia
4. Hypokalemia

Table 3.3 Common causes of chronically delayed gastric emptying

1. Gastric outlet obstruction
2. Postvagotomy
3. Gastric ulcer
4. Scleroderma
5. Dermatomyositis
6. Hypothyroidism
7. Diabetes mellitus
8. Amyloidosis
9. Uremia

Table 3.4 Causes of abnormally rapid gastric emptying

1. Gastric surgery

2. Zollinger–Ellison syndrome

3. Duodenal ulcer

4. Hyperthyroidism

5. Diabetes mellitus

This radionuclide study can detect a bleeding rate as low as 0.1 mL/min. The two common indications for a radionuclide bleeding study are:

1. Suspected acute ongoing or intermittent lower GIB of unknown localization with nondiagnostic endoscopy
2. Follow-up of known bleeding to assess treatment effectiveness

Two radiopharmaceuticals are available for the study of lower GIB: Tc-99m-labeled RBCs and Tc-99m-sulfur colloid:

1. Tc-99m-labeled RBCs is the most commonly used method. Imaging is begun with injection of the radiolabeled RBCs, where dynamic images are taken at a rate of 1 frame/10–60 s. The extravasation manifests as focal activity that appears during the blood pool phase, initially intensifies, and moves anterograde and retrograde on subsequent images (Fig. 3.3). The sensitivity of this method is more than 90%.
2. Tc-99m-sulfur colloid: This study can be performed, in approximately 30 min, in cases of active lower GIB (if no time is available for labeling the RBCs) where time is vital

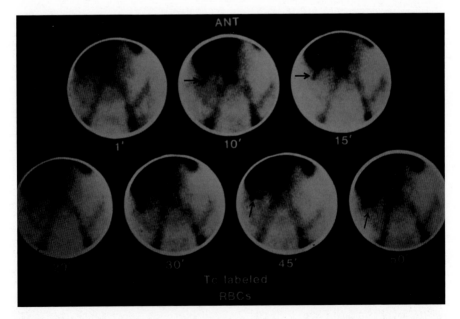

Fig. 3.3 Acute lower GI bleeding as detected on labeled red cell study. Note the extravasated activity that is increasing during the study (*arrows*)

for the management of the patient. This tracer is cleared from the circulation with a half-time of 2.5–3.5 min. By 12–15 min most of the activity is cleared from the vascular system (background), resulting in a high target-to-background ratio. The study is fast and sensitive with quick results, but intermittent bleeding sites may be missed.

The technique of Tc-99m-labeled RBCs is preferred. However, for acute or continuous bleeding, a Tc-99m-SC study may be used. If this is negative or blood loss is known to be intermittent, a labeled RBC study is used since it allows imaging for longer time.

3.7
Diagnosis of Meckel's Diverticulum

Scintigraphy is performed using Tc-99m-pertechnetate (Fig. 3.4), since it is taken up by the ectopic gastric mucosa contained in Meckel's diverticulum. The radiotracer accumulates in and is excreted from the mucus-secreting cells in the ectopic gastric mucosa regardless of the presence of parietal cells.

The patient should be fasting for 4–6 h to reduce gastric secretion passing through the bowel. With Tc-99m-pertechnetate, Meckel's diverticulum appears on imaging at the same time as the stomach and the activity increases in intensity as with the stomach (Fig. 3.5). Pharmacological intervention improves the sensitivity of the study. Cimetidine pretreatment for 2 days before the test enhances gastric uptake and blocks pertechnetate release from the mucosa. Glucagon is given intravenously 10 min after pertechnetate to inhibit peristalsis and delay emptying of gastric contents into the small bowel .

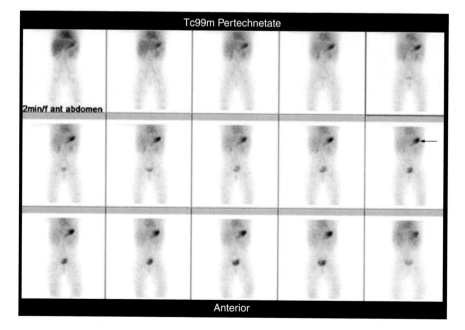

Fig. 3.4 Negative Meckel's diverticulum study. Physiologic update by stomach is seen (*arrow*)

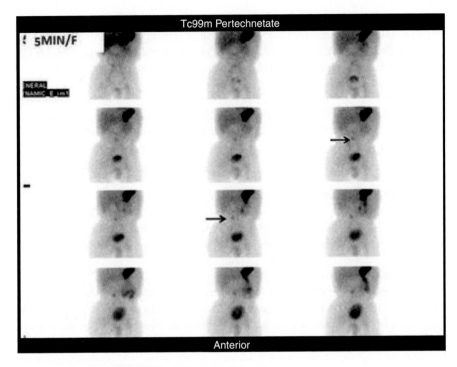

Fig. 3.5 Positive study for Meckel's diverticulum (*arrow*)

The sensitivity of Tc-99m-pertechnetate is more than 85%, but it drops after adolescence because patients who are asymptomatic throughout childhood are less likely to have ectopic gastric mucosa in the diverticulum.

3.8
Diagnosis and Follow-Up of Inflammatory Bowel Disease

Inflammatory bowel disease represents a group of conditions characterized by idiopathic chronic inflammation of the gastrointestinal tract. It includes Crohn's disease, ulcerative colitis, and intermediate colitis.

Crohn's disease is characterized by chronic granulomatous inflammation that can affect the gastrointestinal tract from mouth to anus but most commonly the terminal ileum and cecum, while ulcerative colitis affects the inner layer of the colon with rectal and colonic ulceration. The diagnosis of inflammatory bowel disease (IBD) needs a complex workup and depends mainly on the clinical presentation and biopsy samples taken by colonoscopy. Scintigraphy with radiolabeled leukocytes is able to provide a complete survey of the whole intestinal tract, both the small and large bowel, and detects septic complications successfully. The study is useful in establishing or ruling out IBD in certain patients with

Fig. 3.6 In-111 WBC study showing significant uptake by the colon (*arrow*) indicating active disease

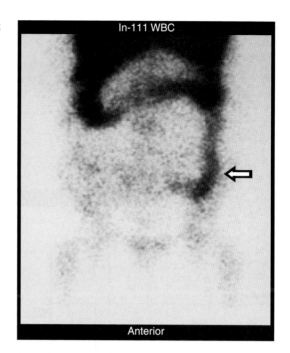

In-111 WBC

Anterior

intestinal complaints, in assessing disease severity (Fig. 3.6), and in the evaluation of extraintestinal septic complications although normal study does not exclude mild inflammation.

Radiolabeled leukocytes studies offer an accepted radionuclide method for imaging inflammation. Because of many advantages of tecnetium-99m (99mTc) over indium-111 (In-111), 99mTc-HMPAO-leukocyte scintigraphy is preferred for the investigation of IBD. The 99mTc-HMPAO-leukocyte scintigraphy technique is highly accurate within the first few hours postinjection. More recently positron emission tomography has been used to assess inflammatory bowel disease.

3.9
Diagnosis of Hepatic Hemangioma

Hemangioma is the most common benign tumor of the liver. Most hemangiomas are of the cavernous type, constituted by dilated nonanastomotic vascular spaces lined by flat endothelial cells and supported by fibrous tissue. Tc-99m-labeled RBC scintigraphy provides the most specific, noninvasive method for making the diagnosis of hepatic cavernous hemangiomas. The use of SPECT provides an advantage over planar only. The study must be interpreted along with the CT scan (Figs. 3.7 and 3.8). If SPECT/CT is available it provides the preferred option.

Fig. 3.7 Negative planar
study for hepatic
hemangioma

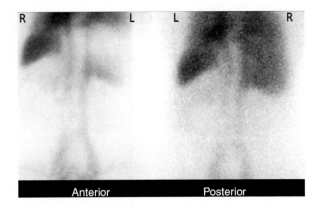

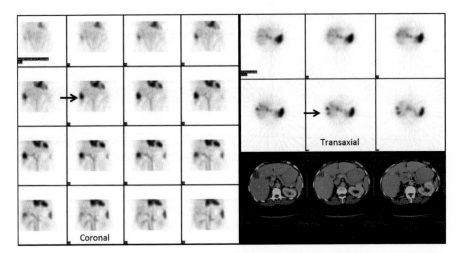

Fig. 3.8 Representative images of a tomographic radionuclide hemangioma study showing a solitary hemangioma (*arrow*) corresponding to the finding on CT but clarifying its nature with high specificity

3.10
Diagnosis of Acute Cholecystitis

Cystic duct obstruction is present in almost all cases of acute cholecystitis. In diagnostically difficult cases, nuclear medicine utilizing Tc99m cholescintigraphy using iminodiacetic acid derivatives is very useful and is the procedure of choice for its diagnosis in such cases. This study carries more than 97% certainty for excluding acute cholecystitis if gall bladder is visualized (Fig. 3.9). It also has a high predictive value for the diagnosis in the proper setting if gall bladder is not visualized (Fig. 3.10).

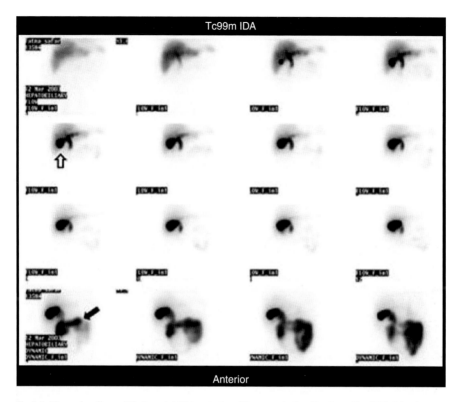

Fig. 3.9 Normal radionuclide hepatobiliary study with prompt visualization of gall bladder (*open arrow*) and intestinal activity (*solid arrow*)

3.11
Diagnosis of Common Bile Duct Obstruction

Radionuclide studies are helpful in many situations to diagnose common bile duct obstruction regardless of the diameter of the duct seen on morphologic studies. Figure 3.11 illustrates an example of obstruction of short duration where liver function has not been affected yet. If it continues the liver function will deteriorate gradually.

3.12
Evaluation of Neonatal Hyperbilirubinemia

Cholescintigraphy utilizing Tc99m IDA (iminodiacetic acid) derivatives is most useful in excluding the diagnosis of biliary atresia with a sensitivity and negative predictive value of virtually 100% when intestinal activity is seen. Patients are typically premedicated with Phenobarbital, 5 mg/kg daily in two divided doses given for 5 days. When intestinal activity is not seen, biliary atresia cannot be excluded (Fig. 3.12).

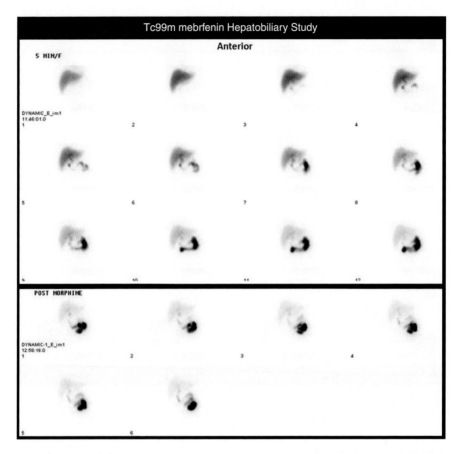

Fig. 3.10 Hepatobiliary study showing nonvisualization of gall bladder during routine study and after low-dose morphine injection in a patient suspected of having acute cholecystitis. The finding indicates obstruction of the cystic duct which indicates acute cholecystitis in the clinical setting of this patient

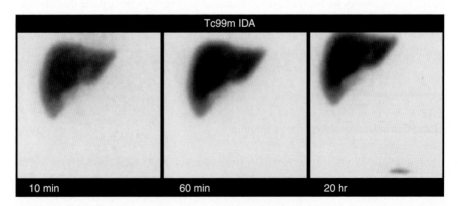

Fig. 3.11 The pattern of acute common bile duct obstruction imaged with Tc-99m IDA. The initial uptake of the liver is adequate with prolonged retention and no evidence of intestinal excretion throughout the study and on delayed image (From Kim [1])

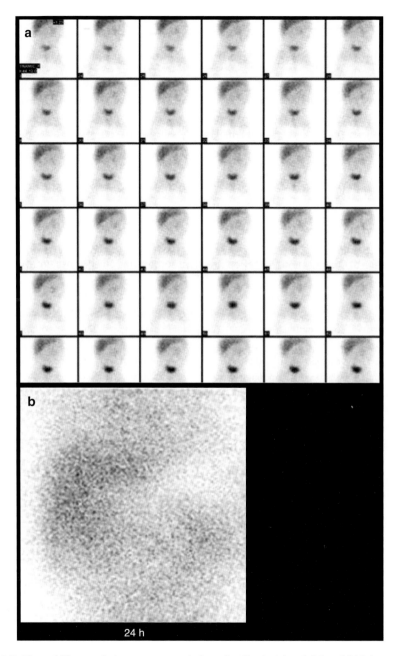

Fig. 3.12 Hepatobiliary study in a neonate carried out for 60 min (**a**) and delayed 24 h image (**b**) illustrating no secretion of activity in the intestine as well as nonvisualization of the gall bladder. Biliary atresia in such case cannot be excluded. However since the function of the liver is adequate biliary atresia is more likely than neonatal hepatitis

3.13
Diagnosis of Hypokinesis Syndrome

Hepatobiliary radionuclide study continues to be very helpful in diagnosing a group of conditions with a common finding of gall bladder hypokinesis. This group includes acalculous cholecystitis, cystic duct syndrome, and others. By using cholecystokinin as diagnostic stimulator during hepatobiliary study, ejection fraction can be determined and low values reflect hypokinesis. This determination helps as an objective evidence in managing these patients since those with chronic acalculous cholecystitis and cystic duct syndrome will benefit from cholecystectomy.

3.14
Evaluation of Complications After Hepatobiliary Surgery and Liver Transplantation

As laparoscopic cholecystectomy has gained popularity and number of liver transplantations has increased. This has led to more utilization of cholescintigraphy for the evaluation of postoperative complications. Bile duct complications include bile leaks, common bile/hepatic duct injuries or strictures, retained biliary calculi, and obstruction. Cholescintigraphy is also useful for assessing the patency of a biliary–enteric bypass or an afferent loop. Liver transplantation has become a popular procedure given the prevalence of hepatitis C and the increasing demand for such life-saving surgery. After transplantation several complications can be evaluated by nuclear medicine procedures particularly biliary leak (Fig. 3.13). If hepatocellular carcinoma is known to be present before transplantation, nuclear medicine helps in preoperative staging and later in restaging the tumor utilizing F-18 FDG-PET studies.

3.15
Protein Loss Study

Protein-losing enteropathy is an uncommon syndrome of excessive loss of protein via the gastrointestinal mucosa. Assessment of protein-losing enteropathy can be conducted scintigraphically (Fig. 3.14) using Tc99m Human Serum Albumen (HAS) which, compare with fecal alpha-1 antitrypsin collection. The study is conducted by imaging the abdomen serially after injection typically at 30 min, 1, 2, and 3 h with further delayed images as needed to look for extravasated activity at sites of intestines. Dynamic images may also be obtained after injection followed by static delayed imaging. The scintigraphic method can also detect esophageal and gastric protein loss. Quantification of protein loss can be performed without the requirement for fecal collection by this method.

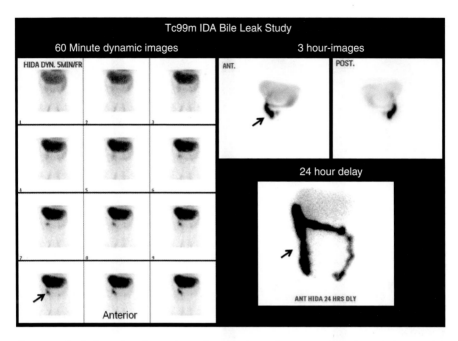

Fig. 3.13 Bile leak study of a patient who underwent liver transplantation 20 days earlier and was referred to rule out possible bile leak. The study shows bile activity early through the study which increased on later images in a linear pattern and appears to be confined within the intestines and colon with no extravasation. Accordingly the study does not show evidence of bile leak

3.16
Scintigraphic Nonimaging Procedures

3.16.1
Carbon-14 Breath Tests

This simple test has been utilized increasingly in recent years in gastrointestinal practice. The test is based on detection and quantitation of radioactive carbon dioxide originating in the stomach or small intestines and exhaled through the respiratory system after being absorbed into the blood stream. The test is useful in the diagnosis of several disease processes, particularly Helicobacter pylori infections, lactose intolerance, and malabsorption due to bacterial deconjugation of bile acids. Nonradioactive Carbon-13 is also used with the same technical concept and accuracy and is replacing C-14 breath test in many facilities.

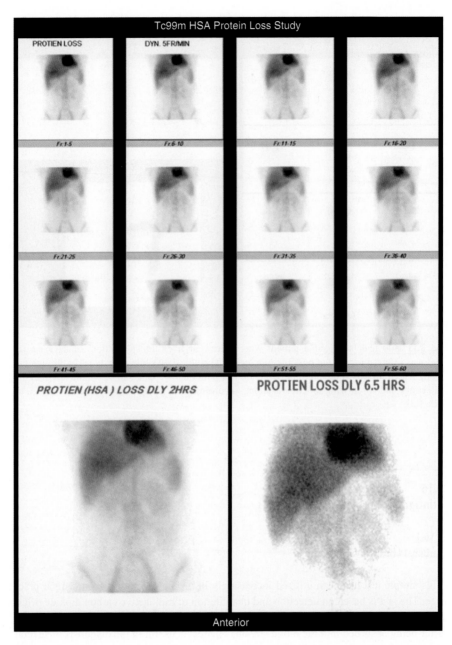

Fig. 3.14 Tc99m Human serum albumin study for protein loss obtained showing dynamic and delayed images with no evidence of extravasated activity indicating no protein loss

3.17
Summary

The scintigraphic methods for gastrointestinal tract diseases are safe, accurate, and well tolerated by adults and children. They are useful and complementary to endoscopy and other imaging modalities in a variety of conditions. They are used in assessment of gastric emptying using Tc99m sulfur colloid. Assessment of cholecystitis, hypokinesis syndrome, biliary obstruction, and biliary leak using Tc99m-IDA derivatives is another important use. Gastroesophageal reflux can be evaluated by oral consumption of the usual diet labeled with Tc99m sulfur colloid. Nuclear medicine imaging techniques allow identification of those patients who are actively bleeding. The demonstration of active bleeding aids in localization of the bleeding site and provides prognostic information. Tc99m-labeled erythrocytes and Tc99m sulfur colloid are two commonly used techniques to detect active bleeding. In addition, Tc99m pertechnetate imaging may be diagnostic of ectopic gastric mucosa in a Meckel's diverticulum as a potential source of bleeding. Intestinal inflammation of inflammatory bowel disease can be evaluated using Tc99m white blood cells. Finally carbon-14 urea breath test is a noninvasive test to detect and follow-up helicobacter pylori infections.

Reference

1. Kim CK, Krynycki BR, Machac J (2006). Digestive system 2: Liver and hepatobiliary tract. In: Elgazzar AH (ed) Pathophysiologic basis of nuclear medicine. Springer, Berlin pp. 437.

Further Reading

Akg NA, Tani Acar E, Taner MS, Zcan Z, Ok E (2005) Scintigraphic diagnosis of protein-losing enteropathy secondary to amyloidosis. Turk J Gastroenterol 16:41–43

Däbritz J, Jasper N, Loeffler M, Weckesser M, Foell D (2010) Noninvasive assessment of pediatric inflammatory bowel disease with 18F-fluorodeoxyglucose-positron emission tomography and computed tomography. Eur J Gastroenterol Hepatol 23(1):81–89

Hassan F, Enezi (2006) Digestive system 1: gastrointestinal tract In: Elgazzar AH (ed) Pathophysiologic basis of nuclear medicine, 2nd edn. Springer, Berlin/New York pp. 395–417

Howarth DM (2006) The role of nuclear medicine in the detection of acute gastrointestinal bleeding. Semin Nucl Med 36:133–146

Warrington JC, Charron M (2007) Pediatric gastrointestinal nuclear medicine. Semin Nucl Med 37:269–285

Zeissman HA (2001) Cholecystokinin cholescintigraphy: clinical indications and proper methodology. Radiol Clin N Am 39:997–1006

Endocrine System

4

Contents

4.1
Introduction

Radionuclide imaging in endocrine diseases has been in clinical application for many years. Over the last six decades changes lead to an increasing number of available radionuclides and radiolabeled compounds for imaging endocrine organ/tissue function. Radionuclide imaging provides functional as well as morphological information on affected endocrine organs especially thyroid, parathyroid, and adrenal disorders. Endocrine nuclear medicine includes not only diagnosis but also internal radionuclide therapy. Recently, radiolabeled peptides have also been used for diagnostic and for therapeutic purposes.

A.H. Elgazzar, *A Concise Guide to Nuclear Medicine*,
DOI: 10.1007/978-3-642-19426-9_4, © Springer-Verlag Berlin Heidelberg 2011

4.2
Thyroid Gland

Nuclear medicine has been successfully used for the diagnosis and treatment of several thyroid disorders. Diagnostically, the common thyroid imaging study using radioiodine or technetium-99m pertechnetate and radioiodine uptake study are routinely used in all hospitals for the diagnosis of and guiding the management of many thyroid conditions. Additionally whole-body imaging study using iodine-131 or iodine-123 is used routinely for thyroid cancer postoperative evaluation and follow-up.

4.2.1
Clinical Uses

- Mass in the neck, tongue, mouth (thyroglossal duct cyst), or chest (substernal thyroid)
- Evaluation of suspected focal (nodules) or diffuse thyroid disease
- Assessment of the function of thyroid nodules identified on clinical examination or by other diagnostic imaging
- Evaluation of the location of functioning thyroid tissue
- Diagnosis and follow-up of thyroiditis
- Preradioiodine treatment of hyperthyroidism
- Suspected occult malignant growth in the thyroid especially in patients with neck irradiation in childhood
- Evaluation of congenital thyroid abnormalities
- Detection and follow-up of thyroid cancer recurrences/or metastases
- Determination of thyroid radioiodine uptake in the following settings:

  1. Differentiating diffuse toxic hyperthyroidism from thyroiditis and thyrotoxicosis factitia
  2. Workup of Grave's disease
  3. Subacute and chronic thyroiditis
  4. Preradioiodine treatment for hyperthyroidism
  5. Postthyroid surgery for differentiated thyroid cancer
  6. Borderline cases of hyperthyroid function by laboratory thyroid function testing

4.2.2
Thyroid Imaging Study

Since the thyroid gland traps iodine from the circulation and uses it to synthesize thyroxin (T4) and triiodothyronine (T3), administration of tracer amounts of radioactive iodine will enable imaging of functional thyroid tissue. Also, pertechnetate is trapped by the thyroid and can be used as an iodine analog for thyroid imaging. If iodine-123 is available it is preferred and is administered orally (3–5 mCi). Imaging is obtained usually 4 h but up to 24 h post administration of radiotracer. When I-123 is not available, the scan is obtained 15 min after the IV injection of 5 mCi of Tc99m-pertechnetate for adults. Anterior and anterior oblique views are obtained whether iodine or technetium is utilized, using a pinhole collimator equipped with 5 mm insert (Fig. 4.1a). Parallel-hole collimator should not

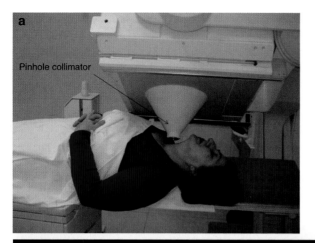

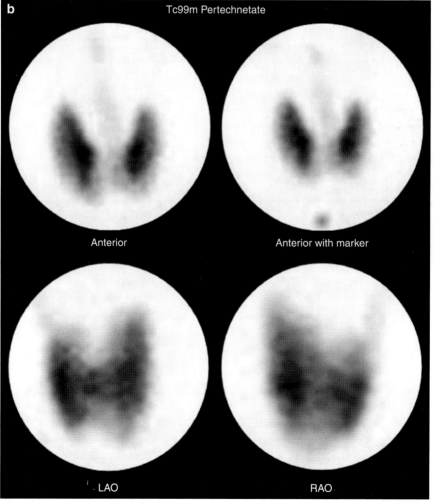

Fig. 4.1 (**a**) Gamma camera equipped with a pinhole collimator (*arrow*) (**b**) Normal thyroid gland

be an option as majority of nodules are missed. Similarly imaging using anterior view only without oblique views results in missing 21% of nodules.

A normal thyroid scan shows homogeneous distribution of ^{123}I or ^{99m}Tc-pertechnetate throughout the gland which appears like a butterfly (Fig. 4.1b). Uptake in the salivary glands and in the soft tissues is noted with ^{99m}Tc-pertechncate and much less with iodine.

Thyroid images should be interpreted in association with clinical and laboratory data (TFT) as well as the result of thyroid uptake especially in cases of hyperthyroidism due to Grave's disease since near normal images can be present in this condition.

Thyroid scan is valuable in suspected nodular disease. It helps determine the number and function of nodules. If nodular disease exists, nodules may appear as solitary or multiple, cold (with decreased to absent uptake) or hot (increased uptake). Figure. 4.2 illustrates an example of a solitary cold nodule while Fig. 4.3 shows a solitary hot nodule.

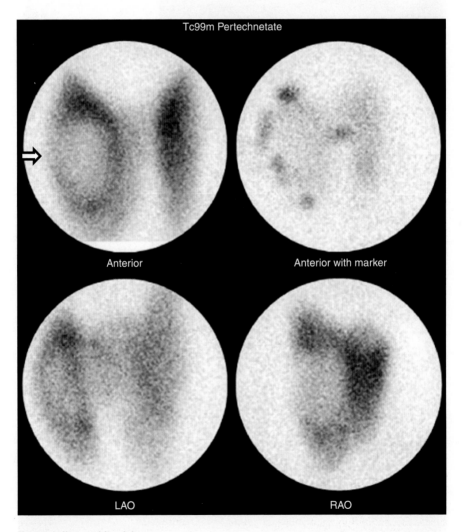

Fig. 4.2 Solitary cold nodule

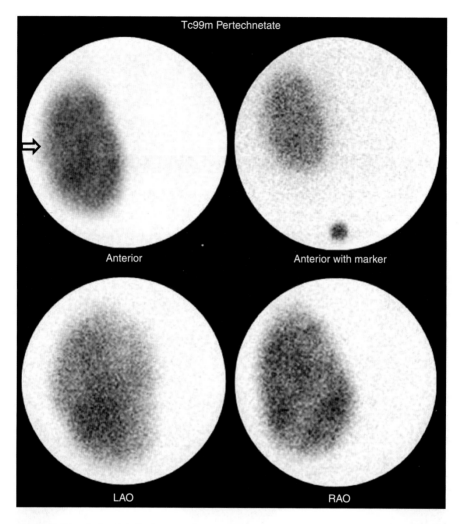

Fig. 4.3 Solitary hot nodule (autonomous)

Multiple nodules are shown in Fig. 4.4. This determination guides further management of nodular disease and estimates along with other parameters the risk of cancer since solitary cold nodule carries 20–25% probability of being malignant while the probability decreases significantly with multiple nodules and when they are hyperfunctioning.

Thyroid scan along with uptake helps differentiate diffuse toxic goiter such as in case of Grave's disease (Fig. 4.5) from thyroiditis (Fig. 4.6) in clinically difficult situations.

4.2.3
Thyroid Uptake Measurement

Normally, the thyroid accumulates a proportion of ingested iodine to synthesize T4 and T3 as needed in the body through feedback mechanisms involving thyroid

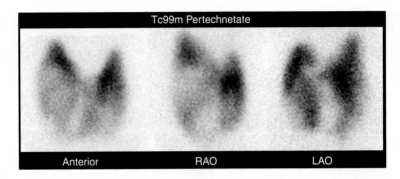

Fig. 4.4 Multinodular gland

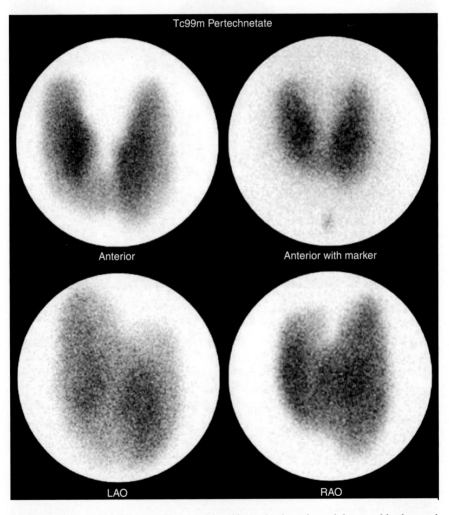

Fig. 4.5 Typical pattern of Grave's disease with uniform gland uptake and decreased background activity in the surrounding soft tissue

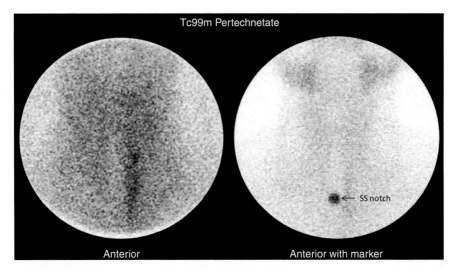

Fig. 4.6 Scintigraphic pattern of thyroiditis where poor uptake and lack of delineation of thyroid gland borders are the typical features

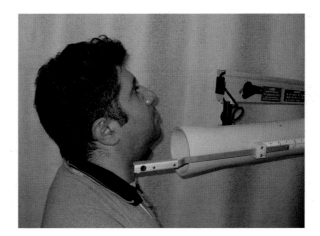

Fig. 4.7 Thyroid probe for radioiodine uptake study

hormones, TSH (thyroid stimulating hormone), and TRH (thyrotropin releasing hormone). Thyroid uptake indicates the level of functional activity of the gland by measuring the trapped proportion of ingested radioiodine at a certain time (2, 4 and/or 24 h). This measurement is useful in assessing the functional status of the thyroid in certain hyperthyroid and hypothyroid states. The study is performed using I-123 or minute activity (7–9 uCi) of iodine-131 and neck counting using a probe (Fig. 4.7). Normal thyroid uptake is 10–35% in most laboratories at 4 and 24 h (range differs according to patient population and technique used and reference values shoud be determined for each laboratory).

4.2.4
Thyroid Cancer Imaging Studies

Some thyroid cancers such as papillary and follicular type, retain the ability to accumulate iodine although to a much lesser extent than normal thyroid tissue. This property is used in the detection of local tumor recurrence as well as distant metastatic spread of thyroid cancer after surgery by administration of iodine and imaging the whole body. This study is used for postthyroidectomy for thyroid cancer for evaluation of regional and distant spread and to detect recurrent functioning cancer in the thyroid bed region or at distant sites. The study is performed after oral administration of small dose of I-131 or higher activity of iodine-123 to the patient who should be fasting for at least 3 h. Images are then obtained 48 h later and if needed at 72 h or later in case of I-131 and 6, 24, and optionally 48 h for I-123. The study is useful to detect residual postoperative tissue, metastases and in the follow-up of therapy. After surgery if no residual thyroid gland nor residual tumor tissue is present, the study will show no foci of abnormal accumulation of radioiodine (Fig. 4.8).

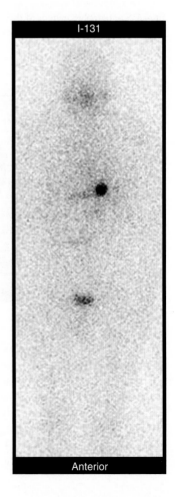

Fig. 4.8 Postoperative I-131 whole-body study with no functioning thyroid tissue in the neck or the rest of the body. Note the physiologic uptake in the salivary glands, stomach, and urinary bladder

Fig. 4.9 I-123 24-h whole-body scan following surgical removal of thyroid gland for differentiated carcinoma. Residual neck thyroid tissue with or without residual tumor is evident (*arrow*)

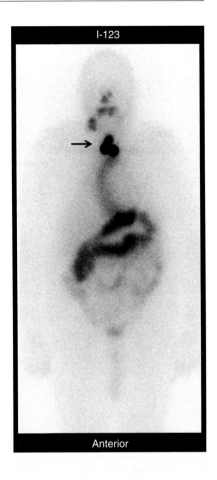

If there are foci of accumulation of the radiotracer they indicate residual thyroid gland and/or tumor tissue in the thyroid bed region (Fig. 4.9) or recurrent or metastatic tumor tissue at distant site(s) if seen on a follow-up study as new finding (Fig. 4.8). It also helps assess the response to radioiodine ablative therapy (Fig. 4.10). Other imaging studies are used particularly when I-123 or 131 study is negative such as thallium 201 and particularly in high-risk patients FDG-PET/CT study (Fig. 4.11).

4.3
Parathyroid Gland

4.3.1
Clinical Uses

1. Preoperative parathyroid localization
2. Intraoperative parathyroid localization

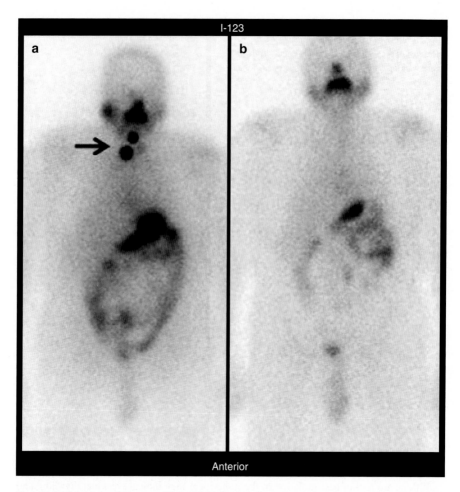

Fig. 4.10 Initial (**a**) and follow-up (**b**) I-123 24-h whole-body scans showing resolution of the neck activity (*arrow*) 1 year after I-131 postoperative ablation

4.3.2
Preoperative Parathyroid Localization

Scintigraphy using Tc99m sestamibi (MIBI) is currently the preferred nuclear medicine method for parathyroid imaging. It is the most sensitive and cost-effective modality for preoperative localization of hyperfunctioning parathyroid tissue. The study is performed by imaging the patient 30 min and 2–3 h postinjection of the radiotracer. Planar, SPECT, and pinhole imaging can all be used for imaging.

Normally Tc99m MIBI is taken by thyroid gland and it clears over time. In the presence of abnormal parathyroid glands the radiotracer is retained in these glands and are seen as foci of tracer accumulation (Figs. 4.12–4.14). This study is beneficial for initial identification of hyperfunctioning glands since it reduces operative time, cost, and

Fig. 4.11 Representative image of an F-18 FDG PET/CT study of a patient with differentiated thyroid cancer showing residual tissue in the nick (*arrow head*)

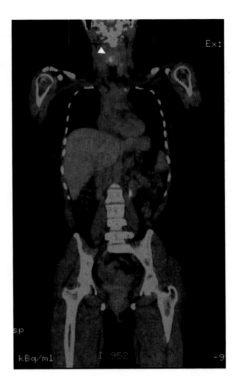

operative failure rates. The sensitivity in localization ranges from 82% to 100% for initial preoperative detection of parathyroid based on the size of the glands. Recently combining SPECT with CT has further improved the localization of parathyroid glands (Fig. 4.15) and has proven the most effective method for localization.

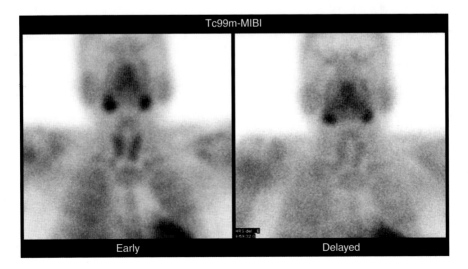

Fig. 4.12 Negative parathyroid study

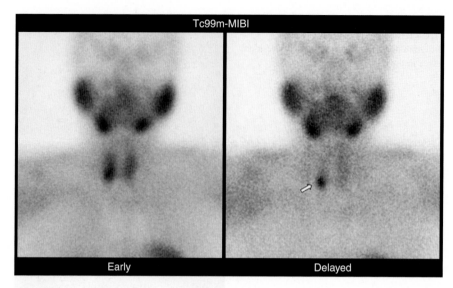

Fig. 4.13 Parathyroid adenoma in the right inferior lobe location (*arrow*)

4.3.3
Intraoperative Parathyroid Localization

Localization using intraoperative gamma probe has recently gained popularity. The patient is injected 2 h before surgery and the probe is used to detect the higher level of activity by the surgeon during surgery.

4.4
Adrenal Gland

Nuclear medicine plays a role in the detection, staging, follow-up, and evaluation of therapy of several adrenal disorders including adrenal cortical and medullary tumors as well as incidental adrenal masses. It can also be used to treat certain adrenal tumors such as neuroblastoma using radioisotopes.

4.4.1
Clinical Uses

1. Diagnosis of certain adrenal cortical disorders such as adenoma and hyperplasia
2. Diagnosis of adrenal medulla disorders particularly neuroendocrine tumors

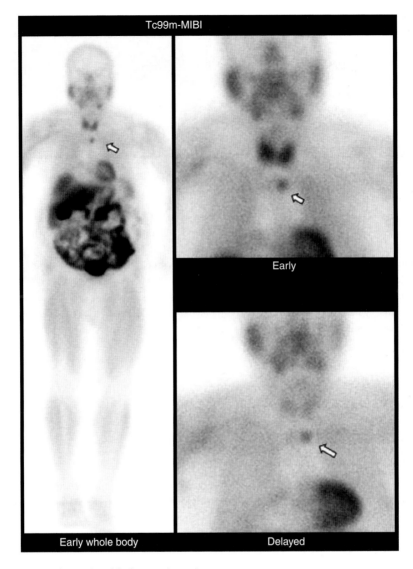

Fig. 4.14 Ectopic parathyroid adenoma (*arrow*)

4.4.2
Adrenal Cortex Disorders

Adrenal cortical imaging study (NP-59 study): NP(^{131}I-6-iodomethyl-19-norcholesterol)-59 is a cholesterol analog that is bound to and transported by low-density lipoproteins (LDL)

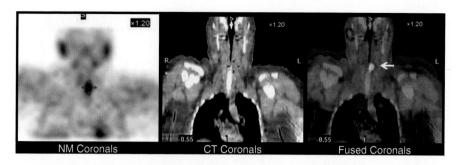

Fig. 4.15 SPECT/CT study showing parathyroid adenoma in the *left* inferior pole location (*arrow*)

to specific LDL receptors on adrenocortical cells. The main value of this study is illustrated in documented cases of adrenal excess secretion and negative or equivocal CT or MRI findings. The scan should be done only on patients with clinically hyperfunctioning adrenal cortex verified by lab results, CT, or MRI.

In primary aldosteronism, early unilateral increased uptake indicates adrenal adenoma, whereas bilateral increased uptake suggests adrenal hyperplasia. Pituitary ACTH-producing adenoma or ectopic ACTH secretion can result in bilateral adrenal hyperplasia.

4.4.3
Adrenal Medulla Disorders

4.4.3.1
Metaiodobenzylguanidine Study

Metaiodobenzylguanidine (MIBG) is a guanethidine analog chemically similar to noradrenaline. It localizes in storage granules of adrenergic tissue (referred to as synaptosomes). Neural crest tumors have these synaptosomes in abundance.

Imaging is performed at 24 and 48 h after injection of ^{131}I-MIBG and at 6 and 24 h after injection of ^{123}I-MIBG. Normally physiologic uptake in the liver, spleen, heart, salivary glands, gut, urinary bladder, and brown fat is noted (Fig. 4.16). Abnormal studies show nonphysiologic accumulation of the radiotracer. The sensitivity of ^{131}I-MIBG in pheochromocytoma (Fig. 4.17) is 80–90% and specificity is more than 90%. Moreover, metastatic and recurrent tumors can also be located. Radiolabeled MIBG imaging is now a well-established examination in the diagnostic evaluation of neuroblastoma. Elevated catecholamine levels are not necessary for its detection by MIBG. The sensitivity of MIBG in neuroblastoma is 91%.

MIBG is localized also in other neuroendocrine tumors to a lesser degree, including carcinoid, medullary thyroid carcinoma, and paraganglioma.

Fig. 4.16 Normal 24 h I-123 MIBG

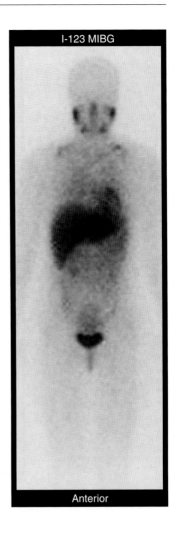

I-123 MIBG

Anterior

4.4.3.2
Indium-111 Tc99m Octreotide Study

In healthy human beings, somatostatin, a natural neuropeptide, is produced in various tissues, including the nervous system, endocrine pancreas, and gastrointestinal tract. Neuroendocrine (including adrenal medulla) and nonneuroendocrine organs have surface receptors that bind to somatostatin. Octreotide, a somatostatin analog with a half-life of 120 min, is used to evaluate the tumors that contain these receptors, in which case it binds to somatostatin receptor subtypes 2 and 5. Among these tumors are pheochromocytoma, neuroblastoma, and paraganglioma, and others including pancreatic tumors and carcinoid.

Fig. 4.17 I-123 MIBG study
showing large
Pheochromocytoma

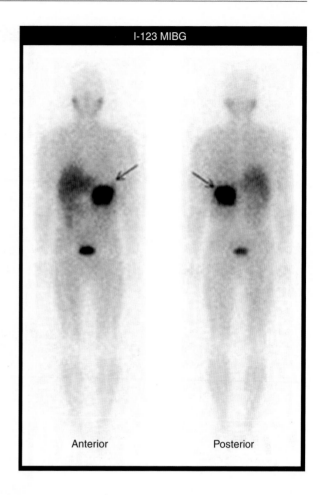

Normally the study shows uniform activity in the liver, spleen, kidneys, gut, and bladder (Fig. 4.18). A focal area of intense early radiotracer uptake is considered to be pathological, indicating primary neoplasm or metastasis (Fig. 4.19). ^{111}In-Tc99m octreotide
scanning is highly sensitive for detecting tumors greater than 1.5 cm.

4.4.3.3
Positron Emission Tomography (PET)

PET has also been used recently to evaluate adrenal masses. Malignant adrenal tumors can
be detected with F-18 FDG PET, but its use in these cases is limited due to the low specificity. C-11 hydroxyephedrine, the first available positron-emitting tracer of the sympathetic
nervous system, was found useful in the detection of pheochromocytomas, with a high

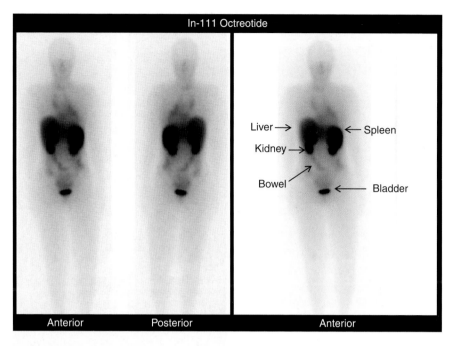

Fig. 4.18 Normal In-111 Octreotide scan (**a**) with an anterior view image illustrating physiologic uptake in labeled organs (**b**)

level of accuracy. Its uptake reflects catecholamine transport and storage and neuronal reuptake. In detecting metastatic pheochromocytomas, F-18-dopamine was found to be superior to I-131 MIBG.

4.5
Summary

Thyroid scan is valuable in suspected nodular disease. It helps determine the number and function of nodules. Thyroid uptake measurement is useful in assessing the functional status of the thyroid in certain hyperthyroid and hypothyroid states. Thyroid cancer whole-body study is used postthyroidectomy for evaluation of regional and distant spread and to detect recurrent functioning cancer in the thyroid bed region or at distant sites as well as in the follow-up. Scintigraphy using Tc99m sestamibi (MIBI) is currently the preferred nuclear medicine method for parathyroid localization as it is the most sensitive and cost-effective modality for preoperative localization of hyperfunctioning parathyroid tissue. Scintigraphic studies are also used to detect and follow up several adrenal disorders particularly neuroendocrine tumors.

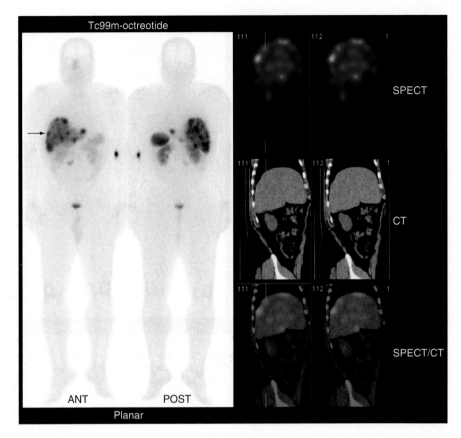

Fig. 4.19 Tc-99 m-octreotide study obtained at 5 h postinjection showing multiple areas of abnormal uptake representing foci of carcinoid tumor in the liver (*arrow*) in the planar images (*left*). SPECT/CT study (*right side panel*) helps better localization of the abnormalities

Further Reading

Elgazzar AH, Gelfand MJ, Washburn LC, Clark J, Nagaraj N, Cumming D, Hughes J, Maxon HR (1995) 1-123 MIBG scintigraphy in adults a report of clinical experience. Clin Nucl Med 20:147–152

Franklyn JA (2009) What is the role of radioiodine uptake measurement and thyroid scintigraphy in the diagnosis and management of hyperthyroidism? Clin Endocrinol 72:11–12

Helal BO, Merlet P, Toubert ME, Franc B, Schvartz C, Gauthier-Koelesnikov H, Prigent A, Syrota A (2001) Clinical impact of (18) F-FDG PET in thyroid carcinoma patients with elevated thyroglobulin levels and negative (131)I scanning results after therapy. J Nucl Med 42:1464–1469

Lumachi F, Tregnaghi A, Zucchetta P, Cristina Marzola M, Cecchin D, Grassetto G, Bui F (2006) Sensitivity and positive predictive value of CT, MRI and I-123 MIBG scintigraphy in localizing pheochromocytomas: a prospective study. Nucl Med Commun 27:583–588

Mettler FA, Guiberteau MJ (2006) Thyroid and parathyroid. In: Mettler FA, Guiberteau MJ (eds) Essentials in nuclear medicine, 5th edn. WB Saunders, Philadelphia, pp 75–100

Okosieme OE et al (2009) The utility of radioiodine uptake and thyroid scintigraphy in the diagnosis and management of hyperthyroidism. Clin Endocrinol 72:122–127

Sarkar S (2006) Thyroid gland. In: Elgazzar AH (ed) Pathophysiologic basis of nuclear medicine, 2nd edn. Springer, New York, pp 209–221

Spies WG, Wojtowicz CH, Spies SM, Shah AY, Zimmer AM (1989) Value of post-therapy whole-body I-131 imaging in the evaluation of patients with thyroid carcinoma having undergone high-dose 1-131 therapy. Clin Nucl Med 14:793

Taillefer R, Boucher Y, Potvin C, Lambert R (1992) Detection and localization of parathyroid adenomas in patients with hyperparathyroidism using a single radionuclide imaging procedure with technetium-99 m-sestamibi (double-phase study). J Nucl Med 33:1801–1807

Wang W, Macapinlac H, Larson SM, Yeh SD, Akhurst T, Finn RD, Rosai J, Robbins R (1999) [18 F]-2-fluoro-2-deoxy-D-glucose positron emission tomography localizes residual thyroid cancer in patients with negative diagnostic 131I whole body scans and elevated thyroglobulin levels. J Clin Endocrinol Metab 84:2291–2302

Soft Tissue Infection and Inflammation

5

Contents

5.1
Introduction

Despite continuous advancements in prevention and treatment methods, infection is still a common problem. The delineation of the site and extent of infection is crucial to the clinical management and for monitoring the response to therapy.

Inflammation is a complex tissue reaction to injury. Injury may be caused not only by living microbes, that is, bacteria, viruses, or fungi, leading to infection, but also by injurious chemical, physical, immunological, or radiation agents.

Acute inflammation is the immediate or early response to injury and is of relatively short duration. It continues only until the threat to the host has been eliminated, which usually takes 8–10 days, although this is variable. Chronic inflammation, on the other hand, is of longer duration and may last from weeks to years. The distinction between acute and chronic inflammation, however, depends not only on the duration of the process but also on other pathological and clinical features. Generally inflammation is considered to be chronic when it persists for longer than 2 weeks.

A.H. Elgazzar, *A Concise Guide to Nuclear Medicine*,
DOI: 10.1007/978-3-642-19426-9_5, © Springer-Verlag Berlin Heidelberg 2011

Acute inflammation is characterized by the following major regional components:

- Local vascular changes including vasodilation, increased vascular permeability, stasis (slowing of circulation), and formation of exudate since increased permeability of the microvasculature, along with the other changes described, leads to leakage with formation of "exudate," an inflammatory extravascular fluid with a high protein content, much cellular debris, and a specific gravity above 1,020. This is the hallmark of acute infection.
- Local cellular events include margination, emigration (leukocytes emigrate from the microcirculation and accumulate at the site of injury), chemotaxis (cells migrate at varying rates of speed in interstitial tissue toward a chemotactic stimulus in the inflammatory focus), and phagocytosis (polymorphonuclear leukocytes and macrophages ingest debris and foreign particles).

Chronic Inflammation on the other hand is characterized by reduction of the number of polymorphonuclear leukocytes but proliferation of fibroblasts with collagen production. Cells will be predominantly mononuclear (macrophages, lymphocytes, and plasma cells). Vascular permeability is also abnormal, but to a lesser extent than in acute inflammation with formation of new capillaries.

5.2
Clinical Uses

Diagnosis, localization, and follow-up of infections.

5.3
Diagnosis of Infection

Diagnosis and localization of infection by clinical and laboratory methods is often difficult. The results frequently are nonspecific and imaging may be needed. Imaging of infection may be achieved by either nuclear medicine or other strictly morphological methods. Several nuclear medicine modalities are used to diagnose and localize soft tissue and skeletal infections. These include [111]In- or tc99m-labeled white blood cells, ^{67}Ga citrate-labeled antibodies such as antigranulocyte antibodies, and F-18-FDG. Plain X-ray, CT, MRI, and ultrasonography are other modalities useful in the diagnosis and localization of both soft tissue and skeletal inflammations. These studies are complementary to the functional modalities of nuclear medicine.

Polymorphonuclear leukocytes migrate to sites of acute inflammation. Radiolabeled white blood cells allow noninvasive detection of sites of occults sepsis or confirmation of the presence of infection in certain preexisting pathological conditions (surgery).

Gallium-67 a radiometal binds to transferrin in plasma and to tranferrin and lactoferrin in inflamed or neoplastic tissue. Early after intravenous administration, Ga-67 is excreted by the kidneys with delayed bowel excretion that can last for several days. Both radiotracers are used to diagnose and localize infection depending on the duration, comorbidities, and whether there are localizing signs.

WBC study is utilized for acute infections, postoperative suspected infections, and inflammatory bowel disease. On the other hand Ga-67 study is more suitable for chronic infections and fever of unknown origin (FUO) of longer duration, certain acute infections, other chronic inflammation (sarcoidosis) and interstitial lung disease, and in suspected infections and inflammatory conditions in patients with HIV.

WBC study is performed after obtaining blood from the patient and labeling it in vitro and reinjection the labeled cells. Images are obtained usually 30 min and 2 h later when tc99m is used for labeling and 4 and 24 h when indium-111 is used. Normally there is uptake in the spleen, bone marrow, liver, and urinary bladder (Fig. 5.1); Ga-67 study is obtained 48 h after injection and can continue for up to 2 weeks. Twenty-four hour images can be used if results needed early but the yield is lower than in later images. Normal gallium study shows uptake in the liver, spleen, salivary gland, bowel, kidneys (early), and bone (Fig. 5.2).

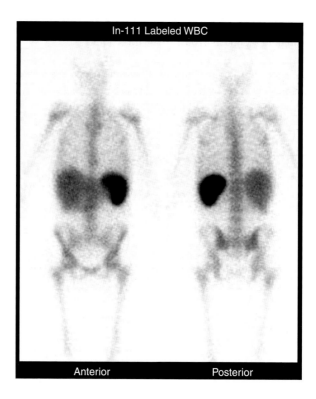

Fig. 5.1 Normal WBC study

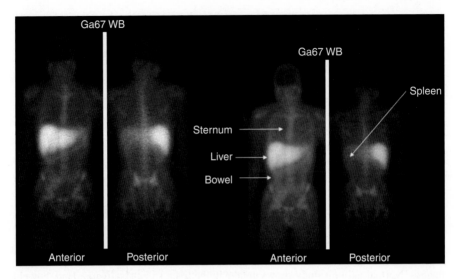

Fig. 5.2 Normal Ga-67 study

5.4
Imaging Diagnosis of Soft Tissue Infections

The strategy for imaging soft tissue infections depends on the pathophysiological and clinical features, including whether localizing signs and symptoms are present and on the location and duration of the suspected infection.

5.4.1
Localizing Signs Present

5.4.1.1
Imaging Abdominal Infections

Rapid and accurate diagnosis of an abdominal abscess is crucial. The mortality from untreated abscesses is high. The mortality among patients treated depends on the time of diagnosis.

Delayed diagnosis is associated with higher mortality in spite of treatment. If localizing signs suggest abdominal infection, morphological modalities, predominantly ultrasound and CT (Fig. 5.3) are used first, depending on the location of suspected infection in the abdomen.

The advantages of these modalities are numerous, but most importantly they provide quick results and adequate anatomical details.

When the results of the morphological modalities are inconclusive, nuclear medicine techniques may be used to detect abdominal infections (Fig. 5.4). The ability to image the entire body is the major advantage of nuclear medicine modalities. Hence radionuclide techniques are often used in cases with no localizing signs.

Fig. 5.3 Periappendicular abscess (*arrow*) on CT scan

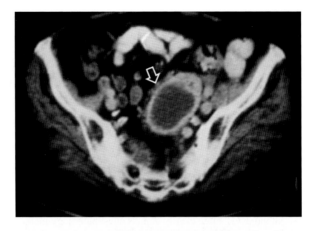

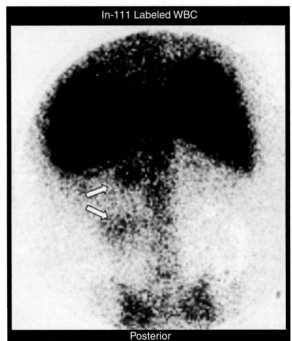

Fig. 5.4 Infected vascular graft on labeled WBC study (*arrows*)

5.4.1.2
Inflammatory Bowel Disease

Upright chest radiography and abdominal series, Barium enema and upper GI, CT scanning, MRI and ultrasonography are the main imaging modalities used for the diagnosis. CT scanning and ultrasonography are best for demonstrating complications such as intraabdominal abscesses and fistulas. Evaluation of the extent of the disease and disease activity is often difficult. A wide variety of functional imaging modalities are available utilizing nonspecific and specific radioactive agents for inflammation. These include Ga67-citrate, radiolabeled autologous leukocytes, antigranulocyte antibodies, and 18F-fluorodeoxyglucose. Scintigraphy using autologous leukocytes, labeled with In111 or

Tc99m, is still considered the "gold standard" nuclear medicine technique for the imaging of infection and inflammation, but the range of radiolabeled compounds available for this indication is still expanding.

Recently, positron emission tomography with F-18-FDE has been shown to delineate various infectious and inflammatory disorders with high sensitivity.

5.4.1.3
Imaging Chest Infections

The role of the chest X-ray cannot be overemphasized. The chest X-ray should be used as the initial imaging modality for most chest pathologies. In many instances, however, an additional modality is needed to evaluate certain chest conditions including infections.

Although CT often clearly depicts chest pathology including infections, ^{67}Ga still is commonly used in such cases. Gallium-67 has also been widely used in AIDS patients to detect PCP. It is highly sensitive and correlates with the response to therapy. Comparing ^{67}Ga, bronchial washing, and transbronchial biopsy in patients with PCP and AIDS, ^{67}Ga and bronchial washing were 100% sensitive compared with 81% for transbronchial biopsy. [67]Ga is also valuable in idiopathic pulmonary fibrosis, sarcoidosis, and amiodarone toxicity. It is also useful in monitoring response to therapy of other infections including tuberculosis (Fig. 5.5).

[111]In WBC imaging is less helpful, as the specificity of abnormal pulmonary uptake (either focal or diffuse) is low. Noninfectious problems that cause abnormal uptake include congestive heart failure, atelectasis, pulmonary embolism, ARDS, and idiopathic conditions.

5.4.1.4
Imaging Renal Infections

The CT scan has good sensitivity and specificity in the diagnosis of renal infections. IVP has a very limited value when the question is urinary tract infection, with a sensitivity of only 25%. Ultrasound has been used frequently to evaluate the kidneys with suspected infections. However the accuracy is inferior to that for cortical scintigraphy which has sensitivity of 86% and specificity of 81%. To date Tc99m DMSA is considered the most sensitive to detect acute pyelonephritis in children.

Positive ultrasonography can obviate the need for DMSA; however, because of a large number of false-negative results with reported sensitivity of 42–58% and underestimation of the pyelonephritis lesions ultrasonography cannot replace tc99m DMSA.

Spiral CT and MRI with contrast have been found to be sensitive in detecting acute pyelonephritis. MRI is not practical because of the cost and the need for sedation for longer period required for imaging.

5.4.2
No Localizing Signs Present

When no localizing clinical signs are present, which is common in cancer and immunosuppressed patients, nuclear medicine procedures are often the imaging modalities chosen. The ability to screen the entire body is particularly important for many such cases.

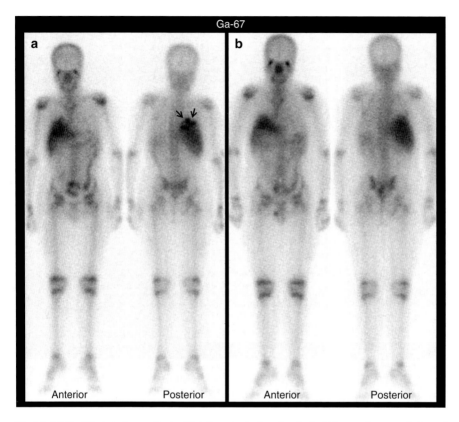

Fig. 5.5 (**a**) Ga-67 study in a patient with tuberculosis showing foci of abnormal accumulation of the radionuclide in the right lung (*arrow*) and a follow-up study (**b**) showing almost complete resolution after therapy

The optimal choice of radiotracer again depends on the duration of infection. Indium-111-labeled white blood cells are the most specific for acute infections (Fig. 5.6), but false-positive results have been reported with some tumors, swallowed infected sputum, GI bleeding, and sterile inflammation. False-negative results have been reported in infections present for more than 2 weeks. Gallium-67 is less specific than labeled WBCs, as it is taken up by many tumors, and by sterile inflammation. However it is more sensitive than labeled WBC in chronic infections (Fig. 5.7). Labeled antibodies and peptides have the potential for a specific diagnosis of infection when the localizing signs are present.

Correlation with morphological modalities after successful radionuclide localization of infection can be of great help. For example, this correlation provides anatomical information prior to surgical interventions.

5.5
Algorithm

Figure 5.8 illustrates simple algorithms for the imaging diagnosis of soft tissue infections utilizing various morphologic and functional modalities.

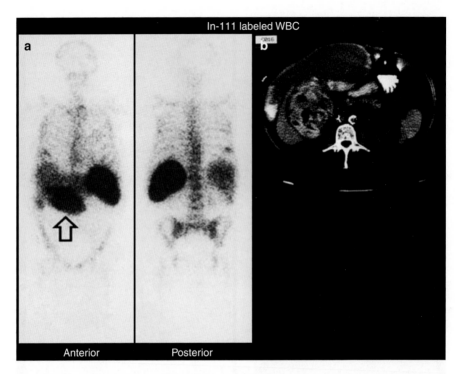

Fig. 5.6 Large abdominal abscess (*arrow*) as seen on labeled leukocyte imaging study (**a**) corresponding to the finding of subsequently obtained CT scan (**b**)

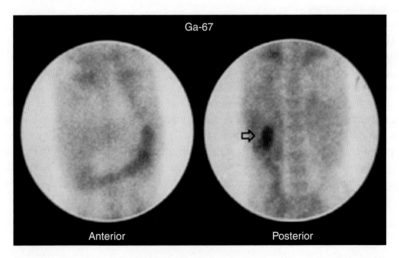

Fig. 5.7 Gallium-67 study of a patient with fever of unknown origin for 6 weeks showing perinephric uptake (*arrow*) representing an abscess

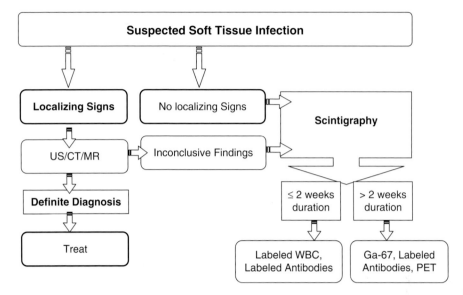

Fig. 5.8 Algorithm for infection imaging

5.6
Summary

Several nuclear medicine modalities are used to diagnose and localize soft tissue and skeletal infections. These include In111-labeled white blood cells, Ga-67 citrate, In111 or Tc99m-labeled monoclonal antibodies such as antigranulocyte antibodies and labeled white blood cells. When there are localizing signs, morphologic modalities such as ultrasonography, CT, and MRI are to be used since they provide fast results and have the advantage of better resolution. When there are no localizing signs or when the results of the morphological modalities are inconclusive, nuclear medicine procedures are the most helpful. When the suspected infection is acute, labeled white cells study is the most suitable whenever possible, while, if the duration of symptoms and signs is more than 2 weeks, or if the infection is believed to be chronic, Ga-67 is more suitable. This is because the number and type of white cells changes when infection becomes chronic. The number of cells decreases and becomes more of mononuclear type which can lead to false-negative results while Ga-67 is not affected.

Further Reading

Elgazzar AH, Elmonayeri M (2006) Inflammation. In: Elgazzar AH (ed) Pathophysiologic basis of nuclear medicine, 2nd edn. Springer, New York/Berlin
Palestro CJ (2009) Radionuclide imaging of infection: In search of grade. J Nucl Med; 50:671–673
Petruzzi N, Shanthly N, Thakur M (2009) Recent trends in soft-tissue infection imaging. Semin Nucl Med 39:115–123

Respiratory System

6

Contents

6.1
Introduction

Respiratory disease is an increasingly significant contributor to morbidity and mortality in the Western world. Lung cancer and chronic bronchitis continue to be major clinical problems. As the population lives longer, there are many older patients with pulmonary disease. These elderly patients are increasingly likely to undergo both emergency and elective surgery, with the associated risks of pulmonary embolism and postoperative infection.

Nuclear medicine has an important role in the diagnosis and in the follow-up of several respiratory diseases. It plays a major role in the diagnosis of pulmonary embolism as well as in the investigation of intrathoracic infection and intrathoracic malignancy. Pulmonary nuclear medicine dates back to Knipping and West in the late 1950s but practically starts

A.H. Elgazzar, *A Concise Guide to Nuclear Medicine*,
DOI: 10.1007/978-3-642-19426-9_6, © Springer-Verlag Berlin Heidelberg 2011

with the successful production of macroaggregated albumin (MAA) by GV Taplin in 1963. This chapter focuses on the major uses of nuclear medicine in respiratory diseases.

6.2
Clinical Uses

The most important uses of nuclear medicine in respiratory system are in the following conditions:

- Suspected pulmonary embolism
- Inflammatory diseases
- Tumors
- Evaluation of alveolar capillary membrane permeability
- Preoperative quantitation of lung function

6.3
Diagnosis of Pulmonary Embolism

The clinical diagnosis of pulmonary thromboembolism is difficult and unreliable, due to the nonspecificity of its symptoms and signs as well as the laboratory and chest x-ray findings. Pulmonary embolism may also be asymptomatic. Only 24% of fatal emboli are diagnosed ante mortem. Data indicate that the mortality of pulmonary embolism is more than 30% if untreated. Promptly diagnosed and treated, emboli have a mortality of 2.5–8%.

Scintigraphy (ventilation/perfusion lung scan) remains the most cost-effective noninvasive screening modality. The major advantages include its ability to provide regional and quantitative information useful for the diagnosis. Additionally it determines the disease severity and monitors its progress. Spiral CT is another complementary modality for diagnosing the condition. Algorithms differ from one institution to another regarding which modality is used first with the other modalities complementing if the initial test cannot solve the clinical question.

Tc99m macroaggregated albumin is used for imaging perfusion. Several agents have been used for ventilation including Xenon 133, Crypton 81, Tc99m DTPA, and Technegas. For proper interpretation of lung perfusion/ventilation study chest x-ray must be available and should be obtained within 12 h of the time of the scans.

Normally perfusion and ventilation studies show uniform distribution of activity throughout the lungs (Fig. 6.1a, b). Typically with pulmonary embolism, perfusion defects are seen with no corresponding ventilation abnormalities or mismatching pattern (Fig. 6.2).

6.4
Pulmonary Sarcoidosis

Sarcoidosis, a multisystem granulomatous disorder, occurs most commonly in young adults, more commonly in blacks and among those who live in temperate areas. The exact etiology is unknown, but it is believed to be due to exaggerated cellular immune response on the part of helper/inducer T lymphocytes to exogenous or autoantigens. The disorder is characterized by the presence of epithelioid granuloma in organs that may lead to fibrosis and organ dysfunction. Lung is involved in more than 90% of cases. Pulmonary sarcoidosis starts as

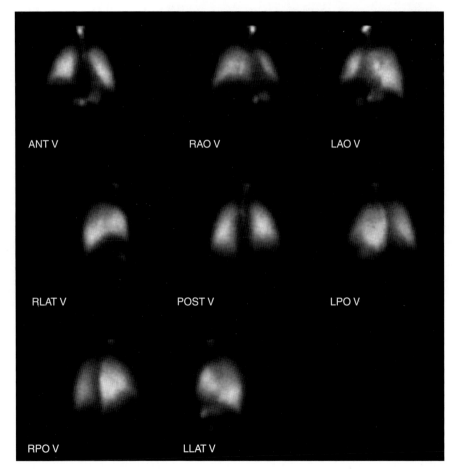

Fig. 6.1 (**a**) Normal Tc99m DTPA aerosol ventilation study. (**b**) Normal Tc99m MAA perfusion study and a diagram illustrating patent pulmonary arteries with no thrombi

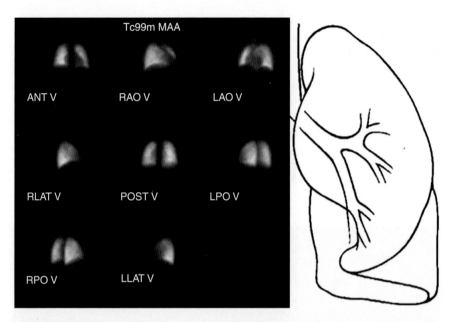

Fig. 6.1 (continued)

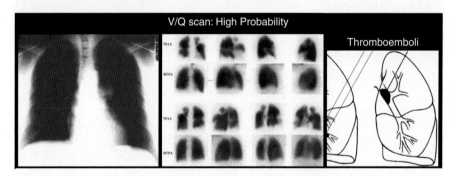

Fig. 6.2 Mismatching (abnormal perfusion and normal ventilation) pattern with no corresponding chest x-ray abnormalities in a case of pulmonary embolism with a diagram illustrating thromboemboli blocking pulmonary arteries preventing blood and radioactive particle from reaching certain segments of the lung causing defects on scan

diffuse interstitial alveolitis, followed by the characteristic granulomas which are present in the alveolar septa and in the walls of the bronchi and pulmonary arteries and veins.

Diagnosis is based on a compatible clinical and/or radiological picture, histopathological evidence of noncaseating granulomas in tissue biopsy specimens, and exclusion of other diseases capable of producing similar clinical or histopathological appearances. Patients with pulmonary sarcoidosis may have no symptoms and discovered by chest x-ray obtained for nonpulmonary reasons. When symptomatic, dyspnea, chest pain, and cough are the most common chest symptoms.

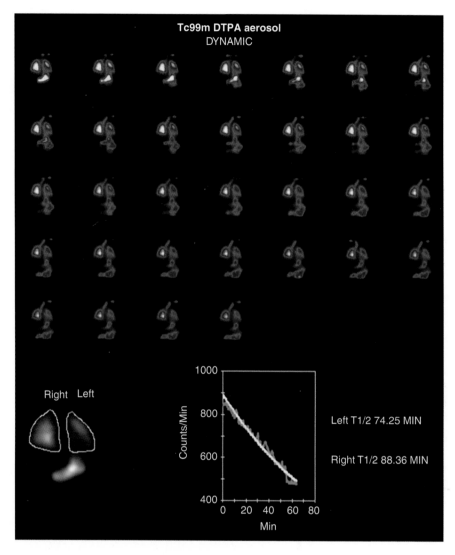

Fig. 6.5 Tc99m DTPA aerosol alveolar–capillary permeability dynamic study (*upper*) with an illustration of regions of interest around the lungs to generate time–activity curves (*lower*) for determination of half clearance time

6.8
Lung Cancer

Lung cancer is currently the leading cause of cancer death among both men and women. Histologically, lung cancer may be squamous adenocarcinoma, small cell carcinoma, adenosquamous carcinoma, and anaplastic carcinoma. The role of nuclear medicine lies in the detection of the primary tumor in certain cases particularly those with solitary lung nodule

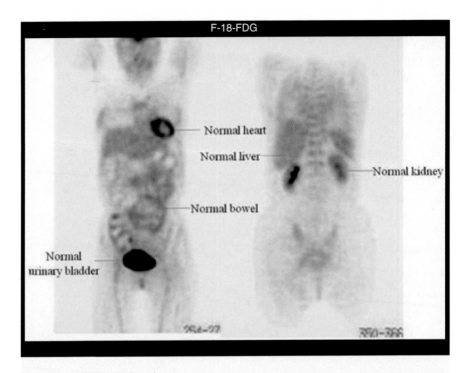

Fig. 6.6 Normal F-18 FDG study

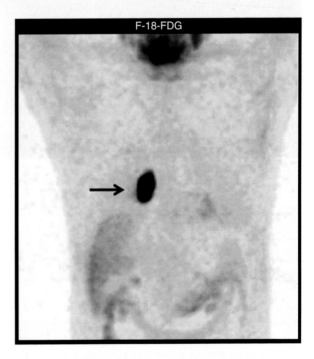

Fig. 6.7 F-18 FDG study
showing a lung cancer
(*arrow*)

on plain x-ray, and more importantly staging of the tumor, and evaluating the response to therapy and in predicting its success. When pneumonectomy is planned for lung cancer, postoperative lung function can be predicted with optimal accuracy by a preoperative perfusion scan in the upright or supine positions providing quantitatively the contribution of various zones to total lung function.

The role of scintigraphy in detecting the primary tumor, staging, evaluating its response to therapy, and locating its metastases involves using several radiopharmaceuticals such as F-18FDG, Ga-67, thallium-201, and Tc99m-sestamibi. PET-FDG is particularly useful in staging the disease and determines the best treatment choice and in the follow-up of the response to therapy (Figs. 6.6 and 6.7).

6.9
Summary

Nuclear medicine contributes significantly in the diagnosis of pulmonary embolic disease. It also helps in the diagnosis of intrathoracic infections and inflammatory conditions and their follow-up. It has a major role in the staging, restaging, and follow-up of intrathoracic malignancies particularly using PET studies.

Further Reading

Elgazzar AH (1997) Scintigraphic diagnosis of pulmonary embolism: unraveling the confusion seven years after PIOPED. In: Freeman LM (ed) Nuclear medicine annual 1997. Lippincott Williams & Wilkins, Philadelphia, pp 69–101

Elgazzar AH, Khadada M (2006) Respiratory system. In: Elgazzar AH (ed) The pathophysiologic basis of nuclear medicine. Springer, Berlin/New York

Leblanc M, Paul N (2010) V/Q SPECT and computed tomographic pulmonary angiography. Semin Nucl Med 40: 426–441

Perrier A, Nendaz MR, Sarasin FP, Howarth NM, Bounameaux H (2003) Cost effectiveness analysis of diagnostic strategies for suspected pulmonary embolism including helical computed tomography. Am J Respir Crit Care Med 167:39–44

Stein PD, Gotlschalk A, Sostman HD, Chenevert TL, Fowler SE, et al. (2008) Methods of prospective Investigation of pulmonary Embolism Diagnosis III (PIOPED III) (2008). Semin Nucl Med 38: 462–470

Stein PD, Sostman HD, Dalen JE, Barley DL, Baj CM, et al. (2011) Controversies in diagnosis of pulmonary embolish Clin. Appl Thromb Hemost 17: 140–149

Contents

7.1
Introduction

Nuclear medicine has an important role in benign and malignant bone diseases. Its role has been expanding significantly particularly in the diagnosis of many benign diseases which may not be detected by morphologic modalities. Table 7.1 summarizes the modalities used in the diagnosis of bone diseases and their main advantages.

Bone scan is the most commonly used nuclear medicine modality for musculoskeletal disorders. To obtain a bone scan the patient is instructed to come well hydrated and is injected with 25 mCi of Tc99m Methylene Diphosphonate (MDP) intravenously, for adults. When multiphase scan is needed, flow phase is acquired as sequential 1 s frames for 1 min. Immediate static image (blood pool) is then obtained for the whole body in the anterior and posterior projections for 5 min (can be regional for the area of interest). Patient is instructed to drink enough fluids (1.5–2 L) and to void frequently. Whole-body delayed static images are obtained 3 h later. Spot images are obtained according to the need for counts based on the location. Images can be obtained later up to 24 h if needed.

A.H. Elgazzar, *A Concise Guide to Nuclear Medicine*,
DOI: 10.1007/978-3-642-19426-9_7, © Springer-Verlag Berlin Heidelberg 2011

Table 7.1 Modalities to image bone

Standard radiographs (plain films)
Useful for fracture, dislocation, bone tumors
Radionuclide bone scan
Allows screening the entire skeleton
Useful for metastatic disease and several benign diseases such as osteomyelitis, occult fractures, avascular necrosis, complex regional pain syndrome, and heterotopic bone formation
Computed tomography (CT)
Useful for assessing cortical disruption
Magnetic resonance imaging (MRI)
Useful for assessing marrow involvement; vertebral metastases, vertebral osteomyelitis diabetic foot infection, osteomyelitis
Soft tissues around joints (collateral ligaments, menisci in knee)

Normal scan (Fig. 7.1) should show symmetric uptake. In general symmetry should be considered normal till otherwise proven and any asymmetry should be considered abnormal till proven otherwise. Certain areas are normally known to show relatively increased uptake in both pediatric and adult age-groups due to higher bone turnover.

7.2
Clinical Uses

- Non-neoplastic diseases
  - Infection: diagnosis and follow-up of skeletal infections
  - Vascular diseases: diagnosis of avascular necrosis
  - Traumatic diseases and related conditions: diagnosis of radiologically occult fractures
  - Metabolic diseases: Diseases such as Paget's disease and renal osteodystrophy
- Neoplastic diseases
  - Primary tumors: limited role, assessing multiplicity and metastases
  - Metastatic bone disease: very sensitive ways to detect bone metastases in many malignancies as well as their follow-up

7.3
Non-neoplastic Disease

7.3.1
Imaging of Skeletal Infections

Several imaging modalities are now being utilized for the diagnosis of osteomyelitis, including standard radiography, computerized tomography (CT), magnetic resonance imaging (MRI), and nuclear medicine techniques. The choice of modality depends on

Fig. 7.1 Normal bone scan

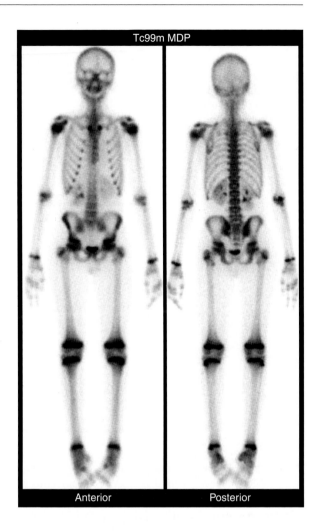

clinical presentation, duration of symptoms, site of suspected infection, previously known underlying pathology (such as fracture or tumor), and other factors.

7.3.1.1
Acute Osteomyelitis

Standard radiographs are not sensitive for early detection of osteomyelitis, as the changes are evident only after 10–21 days from the time of infection. Bone scintigraphy is very sensitive in the early diagnosis of osteomyelitis and can show the abnormality as early as 24 h after infection. Typically, there is focally increased flow, blood pool activity, and delayed uptake (Fig. 7.2). When the bone has not been previously affected

Fig. 7.2 Three phase bone
scan illustrating focally
increased flow (**a**) blood pool
(**b**) and corresponding
increased uptake on delayed
image (**c**) in a case of acute
osteomyelitis

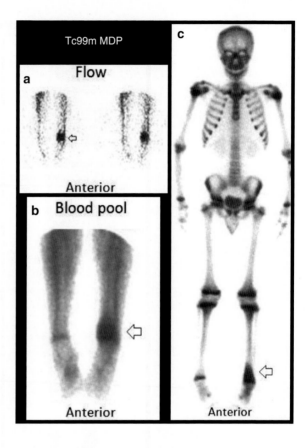

by other pathological conditions (nonviolated), the bone scan has high accuracy and is
a cost-effective modality for diagnosis of osteomyelitis with both sensitivity and specificity of 90–95%.

If bone has been affected by a previous pathology (violated), particularly after orthopedic
surgical procedures, the bone scan will still be highly sensitive but the average specificity is
only approximately 34%. In such situations, unless the bone scan is unequivocally negative,
an additional modality should be used, particularly leukocytes labeled with ^{111}In-oxine or
[99m]Tc-hexamethyl propylene amine oxime (HMPAO). Overall, ^{111}In-leukocyte studies have a
sensitivity of approximately 88% and a specificity of 84% for osteomyelitis.

This modality is particularly useful for excluding infection in previously violated bone
sites such as in postsurgical and post-traumatic conditions as well as diabetic foot skeletal
infections. Combined labeled-leukocytes and bone scans have a better accuracy than
labeled-leukocyte scans alone and can help to localize abnormal foci. Using SPECT/CT is
even more accurate particularly in certain sites such as the foot.

Since labeled-leukocyte scans show uptake by active bone marrow, it may be difficult
to differentiate this normal marrow uptake from abnormal uptake due to infection.
Furthermore, surgical procedures may alter the bone marrow distribution significantly.
Bone marrow scans using ^{99m}Tc-sulfur colloid or nanocolloid may improve the specificity
of such studies.

Labeled antibodies such as ^{111}In- or ^{99m}Tc-labeled human nonspecific polyclonal antibodies and antigranulocyte antibodies are other nuclear medicine methods but did not achieve universal acceptance.

7.3.1.2
Chronic and Vertebral Osteomyelitis

The radiological diagnosis of chronic active osteomyelitis is neither sensitive nor specific, while bone scintigraphy is very sensitive but not specific. This low specificity is due to the chronic bone repair that is associated with increased bone metabolism and increased uptake on bone scan in the absence of active infection. It is therefore difficult to differentiate healing from chronic active disease, although increased activity on all phases of the bone scan is suggestive of chronic active disease. The bone scan, accordingly, cannot confirm the presence of active disease, but a negative scan excludes it.

Gallium-67 citrate imaging is more specific than bone scanning for chronic osteomyelitis. False positives still occur in conditions such as healing fractures, tumors, and noninfected prostheses. Combined ^{99m}Tc-MDP and ^{67}Ga scans can be helpful in making the diagnosis of active disease. Recently, PET has been found useful to assess the activity of chronic osteomyelitis.

Signs and symptoms of vertebral osteomyelitis are usually vague and insidious and thus the diagnosis and treatment may be delayed. Plain x-rays are neither sensitive nor specific for the diagnosis of vertebral infection. The bone scan may be sensitive but it is not specific.

Computed tomography scan is quite sensitive for vertebral osteomyelitis but, like the bone scan, it is not specific. However, CT is used to guide needle biopsy.

Magnetic resonance imaging, on the other hand, is both sensitive and specific for vertebral osteomyelitis. Indium-111-labeled leukocyte scans are not generally useful in the diagnosis of vertebral osteomyelitis as the images may show normal or decreased uptake and accuracy is low. Because the diagnosis of vertebral osteomyelitis is often delayed, most infections are chronic in nature, which explains the low sensitivity of ^{111}In-labeled leukocytes in its diagnosis. Gallium-67 has a sensitivity of 90% and a specificity of 100% when combined with ^{99m}Tc-MDP.

MRI is as accurate as combined ^{99m}Tc and ^{67}Ga isotope scanning. FDG-PET may be useful in excluding infection when other modalities are equivocal.

7.3.1.3
Infectious (Septic) Arthritis

Bone scan is useful in differentiating osteomyelitis from septic arthritis. In septic arthritis there is increased flow and blood pool activity with either normal delayed images or there is mildly increased uptake that is periarticular, uniform, and confined to the joint capsule. It has been reported that identifying joint involvement and distinguishing bone from joint infection can be achieved in up to 90% of cases using bone scintigraphy.

To simplify the utilization of the many imaging modalities a suggested algorithm for the diagnosis of skeletal infection is shown in Fig. 7.3.

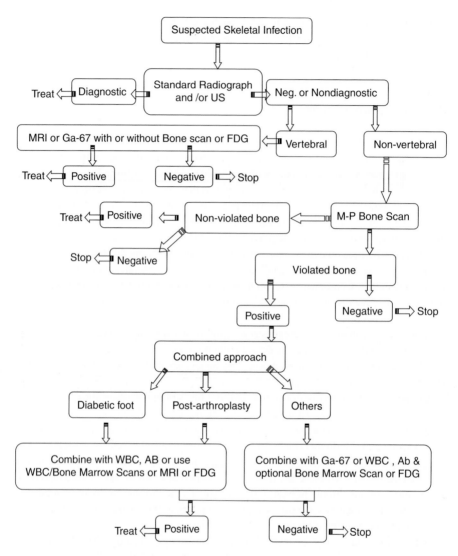

Fig. 7.3 Simple guide for imaging of skeletal infections

7.3.2
Avascular Necrosis (Osteonecrosis)

Avascular necrosis of bone results from imbalances between the demand and supply of oxygen to osseous tissues. There are many causes for osteonecrosis (Table 7.2). In some cases the underlying cause cannot be determined and in this situation the term primary, idiopathic, or spontaneous osteonecrosis is used.

Following the interruption of blood flow, blood forming and mesenchymal cells of the marrow as well as primitive osteoblasts are involved first and die 6–12 h after the

Table 7.2 Causes of avascular necrosis of bone

1. Trauma (e.g., fracture or dislocation)
2. Hemoglobinopathies (e.g., sickle cell anemia)
3. Exogenous or endogenous hypercortisolism (e.g., corticosteroid medication, Cushing's syndrome)
4. Renal transplantation
5. Alcoholism
6. Pancreatitis
7. Dysbaric (e.g., Caisson disease)
8. Small vessel disease (e.g., collagen vascular disorders)
9. Gaucher's disease
10. Hyperuricemia
11. Irradiation
12. Synovitis with elevation of intra-articular pressure (infection, hemophilia)
13. Idiopathic (spontaneous osteonecrosis) including Legg-Calvé-Perthes disease in pediatrics

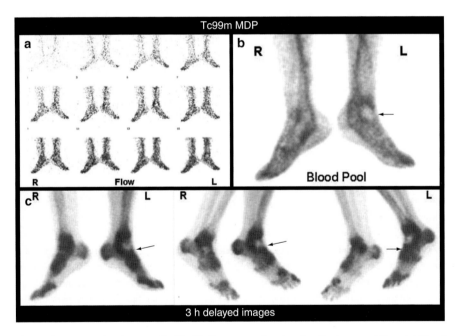

Fig. 7.4 Representative images of a 99mTc Bone scan showing focally decreased flow (**a**) blood pool activity (**b**) and delayed uptake (**c**) in a case of acute avascular necrosis of the left navicular bone (*arrows*)

interruption of the blood supply. Bone cells including osteocytes and mature osteoblasts die 12–48 h later, followed by the fat cells, which are most resistant to ischemia and die 2–5 days after the interruption of blood flow. The different scintigraphic patterns of femoral head avascular necrosis are correlated with the sequence of pathological events. In early stage uptake on bone scan varies and eventually a cold area (absent uptake) develops (Fig. 7.4).

Fig. 7.5 Healing phase of avascular necrosis with a rim of increased uptake around a central focus of decreased uptake in the left femoral head (*arrow*)

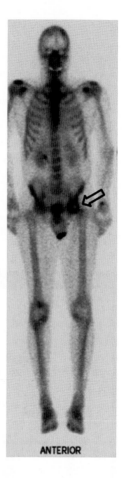

ANTERIOR

Later on, the reparative process is initiated and carried out by neovascularization through the collateral circulation advancing from the periphery of the area of necrosis or by recanalization of occluded vessels. This phase is characterized scintigraphically by increased technetium uptake starting at the boundaries between the site of necrosis and the normal tissue beginning in 1–3 weeks (Fig. 7.5). This increased uptake eventually will advance around a central photopenic area and may last for several months. As the reparative process is completed, uptake returns to normal. However, in cases with bone collapse increased uptake may persist indefinitely.

7.3.3
Trauma and Related Conditions

Trauma to the musculoskeletal system may affect bone, cartilage, muscles, and joints. To each of these structures, trauma may cause immediate damage and late changes. The role of scintigraphy in fracture diagnosis is limited to those cases of radiologically occult fractures, fractures of the small bones of the hands and feet including the underrecognized condition of Lisfranc fracture and stress fractures. It is also useful for early detection of heterotopic bone formation and to determine the appropriate time for surgical removal by determining maturity.

7.3.3.1
Fractures of Small Bones

Bone scintigraphy is particularly important in the diagnosis of radiologically occult fractures of small bones of the hands and feet (Fig. 7.6). Pinhole imaging can be of additional help in localizing the abnormalities.

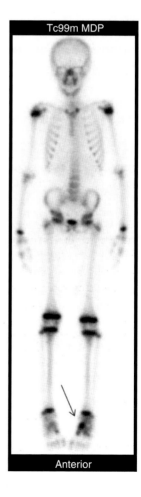

Fig. 7.6 Fracture of the left navicular bone (*arrow*)

7.3.3.2
Stress Fractures

Stress fractures are due to repeated stress, each episode of which is less forceful than required to fracture the bony cortex. The stress fracture is not as thought due to repeated traumatic microfractures due to the stress. It is a focal area of increased bone turnover secondary to the repeated stress. If this occurs in normal bones, the resulting fractures are called fatigue fractures, while if they occur on abnormal bones, as in osteoporosis, they are termed insufficiency fractures.

Bone scintigraphy is much more sensitive than standard radiographs in detecting stress fractures. Fatigue fractures are common in athletes, military personnel, and dancers. If scintigraphy is performed in the acute phase of less than 4 weeks, the flow and blood pool images show increased activity (Fig. 7.7). Later, only delayed uptake will be seen. The delayed uptake is typically focal or fusiform, involving less than one-fifth of the bone. This is different from the pattern of a shin splint, which is another consequence of stress and occurs in the same patient population as fatigue fractures. Shin splints typically show normal flow and blood pool images, with an elongated linear pattern of increased uptake on delayed images. They are most commonly found in the tibiae (Fig. 7.8) and may coexist with fatigue fractures in the same patient. The pattern seen with shin splints is due to subperiosteal bone formation.

7.3.3.3
Lisfranc's Fracture (Tarsometatarsal Fracture)

Bone scan is a sensitive modality to detect this condition which is difficult to detect on plain film and can be frequently missed. On bone scan increased perfusion and delayed uptake are noted at the site of tarsometatarsal joints (Fig. 7.9).

7.3.3.4
Spondylolysis

Spondylolysis is a condition in which there is a loss of continuity of bone of the neuro-arch of the vertebra due to trauma, or more likely to stress. The diagnosis is principally

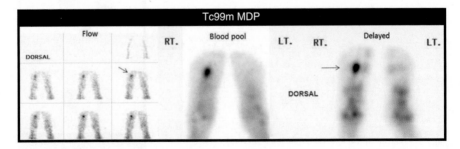

Fig. 7.7 Pattern of stress fracture on bone scan

Fig. 7.8 The linear uptake of shin splints (*arrow*)

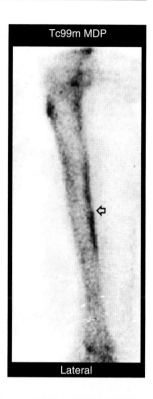

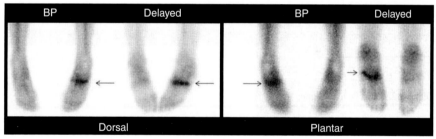

Fig. 7.9 Lisfranc fracture on bone scan. There is increased activity on blood pool images and uptake on delayed images at the side of tarsometatarsal joints (*arrows*)

radiological, and scintigraphy is reserved for detection of radiologically occult stress changes and for assessing metabolic activity of the condition (Fig. 7.10).

7.3.3.5
Growth Plate Injury

Scintigraphic imaging complements anatomic studies by reflecting the physiological status of the growth plate and has the advantage of quantitation. It can also detect the abnormalities earlier than morphologic modalities and can help particularly in detecting segmental growth plate arrests that are difficult to determine by these modalities.

Fig. 7.10 Planar (**a**) and
selected cuts of tomographic
bone imaging study (**b**, **c**) of
a 17-year-old male
complaining of back pain.
The study shows findings of
spondylolysis affecting
L-4/L-5 seen clearly on
tomographic study (*arrows*)
but not so on planar image

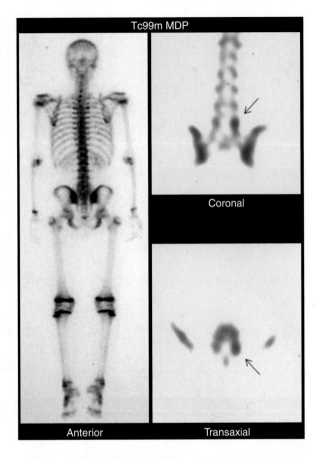

7.3.3.6
Complex Regional Pain Syndrome-1(CRPS-1)

Complex regional pain syndrome Reflex Sympathetic Dystrophy is a clinical syndrome characterized by pain, hyperalgesia, edema and abnormal vasomotor activity, joint stiffness, regional osteopenia, and dystrophic soft tissue changes.

The most common synovial histopathological changes are proliferation of synovial cells, subsynovial fibrosis, and vascular proliferation.

Vascular changes can be demonstrated on ^{99m}Tc diphosphonate blood pool images, which show increased periarticular activity. The proposed pathophysiological mechanism of the condition is related to an initial triggering injury most commonly trauma causing an imbalance between the nociceptors and the autonomic nervous system (sympathetic and parasympathetic) to the affected area. As a result, vasomotor disturbances take place with vasodilatation as a prominent feature, leading to increased blood flow to the synovial and osseous tissues. The synovium reacts with cell proliferation and eventually secondary fibrosis. The adjacent bone undergoes increased turnover locally, with some resorption.

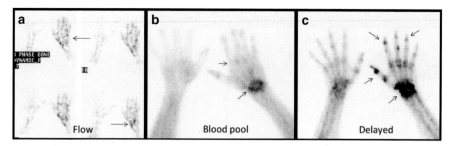

Fig. 7.11 Acute complex regional pain syndrome type I in a 67-year-old male with cerebrovascular accident and right-sided hemiplegia. The patient was complaining of progressive right hand pain, burning & swelling for 10 days not responding to analgesia. The study shows increased flow (**a**) blood pool (**b**) and delayed uptake (**c**) in the right hand in a periarticular pattern (*arrows*)

The scintigraphic pattern depends on the duration or stage of the disease. In the first or acute stage (20 weeks), all three phases of bone scan show increased activity (Fig. 7.11). After 20 and up to 60 weeks during the dystrophic phase, the first two phases are normalized, while the delayed-phase images show increased periarticular uptake. After 60 weeks (atrophic phase), the flow and blood pool images show decreased perfusion, with normal uptake on delayed images.

Bone scintigraphy can be used not only to help in the diagnosis but also to monitor the disease with treatment.

7.3.3.7
Heterotopic Bone Formation

Heterotopic bone formation is a common condition most frequently following trauma including surgery. It is a formation of bone in sites that do not normally contain bone. It is believed to be due to transformation of mesenchymal cells to bone forming cells. Bone scintigraphy is useful for early detection of heterotopic bone formation and to determine the appropriate time for surgical removal by determining maturity (Fig. 7.12).

7.3.4
Metabolic Bone Diseases

Metabolic bone diseases are common and may be difficult to diagnose on the basis of clinical and radiologic findings. Metabolic bone disease is usually linked to alterations of the calcium metabolism. Increased rates of bone turnover are present in most metabolic bone disorders often associated with decreasing calcium content of the affected bone. This explains why most metabolic disorders result in generalized increased radiopharmaceutical uptake on bone scan, reflecting this increased bone turnover (Fig. 7.13).

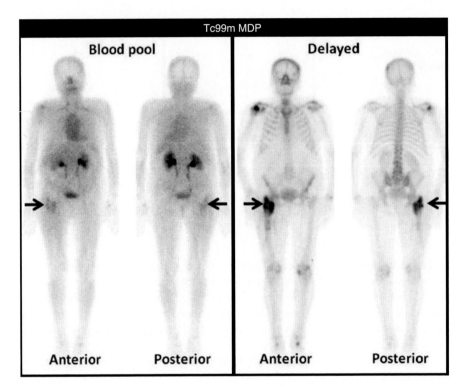

Fig. 7.12 A case of immature heterotopic bone formation with increased blood pool activity and corresponding delayed uptake at the site of soft tissue bone formation (*arrows*)

Bone scintigraphy is helpful in detecting and follow-up of several metabolic bone diseases such as Paget's disease, renal osteodystrophy, and fibrous dysplasia.

7.4
Diagnosis of Neoplastic Bone Disease

Evaluation of bone tumors, whether being primaries or the more commonly occurring metastases, involves use of several imaging modalities. Generally, functional nuclear medicine procedures have a limited role in evaluation of primary bone tumors though they are substantially useful in detecting metastasis, following up the response to therapy and estimating prognosis. CT scan and MRI are often complementary and are particularly useful in primary bone tumors. MRI, however, is superior in evaluating the regional extent of several primary tumors and detecting involvement of bone marrow. Nuclear medicine procedures that involve imaging of bone tumors utilize 99mTc MDP, I-123 or I-131 MIBG,

Fig. 7.13 A case of renal osteodystrophy illustrating the scintigraphic pattern of metabolic bone disease. Note the prominent uptake in the calvarium, mandible, costocondral junctions, long bones, and spine

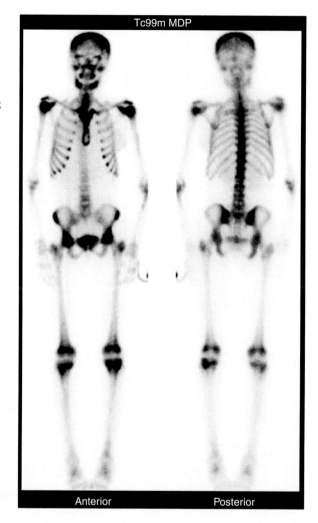

Ga-67, Thallium-201, 99mTc MIBI, and PET imaging. The following discussion presents the role of functional imaging in correlation with structural modalities in the diagnosis and management of primary and metastatic bone tumors.

7.4.1
Imaging of Primary Bone Tumors

Functional nuclear medicine imaging plays a minor role in evaluating the local extent of the primary bone tumors (Fig. 7.14). However, it helps in staging the tumor by identifying

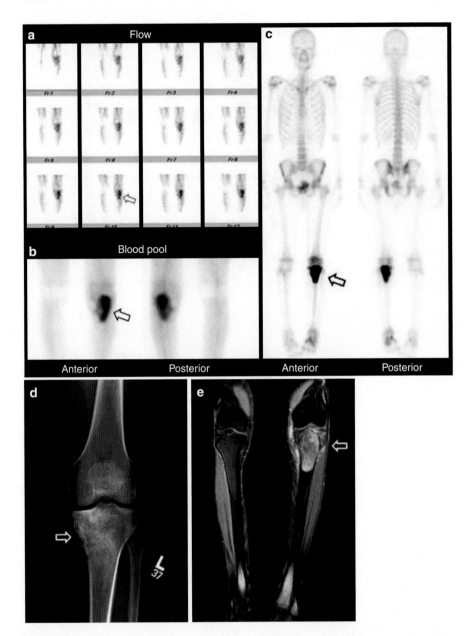

Fig. 7.14 A 14-year-old male with pain and swelling of the left upper leg proven later to be osteogenic sarcoma. Bone scan shows hypervascularity (**a**, **b**) and intensely increased delayed uptake (**c**) corresponding to the x-ray (**d**) and MRI (**e**) findings. Note the mildly diffuse increased uptake in the bones of the left lower extremity due to disuse. No distant metastases. Note the outlines of the tumor on MRI images which is superior to bone scan in regional staging of the tumor

other sites of involvement and in evaluating the response to chemotherapy. PET-FDG particularly plays an important role in evaluating prognosis and response to therapy.

7.4.2
Imaging of Metastatic Bone Disease

Nuclear medicine plays a very important role in evaluating bone metastases of different extraosseous primary tumors. Bone metastases are common at the time of the diagnosis and follow-up of many primary tumors (Table 7.3).

In general, four main modalities are routinely utilized clinically to assess bone, the third most common site of metastatic diseases, for existence of metastatic lesions. These modalities include standard radiography, CT scan, bone scintigraphy, and MRI. Bone scan is the most widely used modality and is the most practical and cost-effective screening technique for assessing the entire skeleton. In addition, bone scan is very sensitive in detecting the disease. However, there is a variable false-negative rate in assessing lesions in certain locations particularly in the spine and in those confined to bone marrow. MRI has been found to detect more vertebral metastases than bone scan. PET is increasingly evaluated for detection of bone metastases and the initial experience is promising, and was shown by several studies to be more sensitive than bone scan, though not fully supported.

7.4.2.1
Appearance of Metastases on Bone Scan

Typical Pattern

The most common and typical pattern of bone metastases is that of multiple randomly distributed foci of increased uptake, usually in the axial skeleton following the distribution of bone marrow including the shoulder girdle with relatively less extensive involvement of the ribs (Fig. 7.15). Metastases to the peripheral bones of the extremities are rare.

Table 7.3 Bone metastasis and tumor type

Tumor	Incidence (%)
Myeloma	70–95
Breast	50–75
Prostate	50–75
Thyroid	40–60
Lung	30–40
Melanoma	14–45
Osteosarcoma	25
Renal	20–25

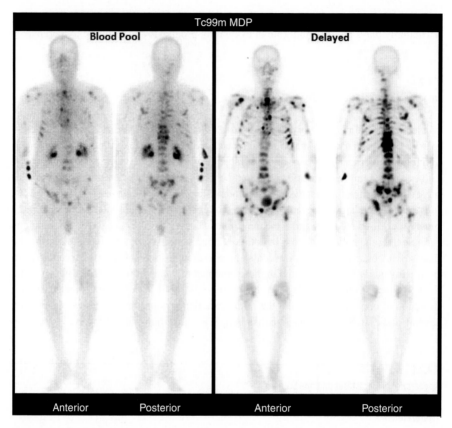

Fig. 7.15 Typical metastatic bone disease pattern on bone scan with randomly distributed foci of increased uptake affecting the axial skeleton

Atypical Patterns

Solitary Lesion

Solitary metastasis occurs in axial and in appendicular skeleton in variable percentages of cancer patients. These lesions are commonly asymptomatic and not suspected clinically. Less than half of these lesions are present on x-rays. These facts further emphasize the importance of obtaining a bone scan of the entire skeleton in patients with cancer. The incidence of malignancy in solitary lesions (Fig. 7.16) varies with the location. The incidence is highest in the vertebrae and low in the skull and extremities.

Fig. 7.16 Solitary bone lesion on bone scan (*arrow*) proven to be metastasis

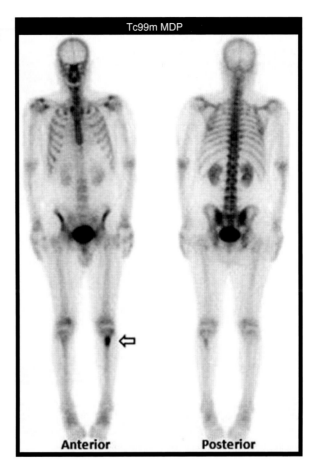

Cold Lesions

Cold lesions on bone scan (Fig. 7.17) are seen in aggressive tumors, commonly, multiple myeloma and renal cell carcinoma.

Diffuse Pattern

The entire axial skeleton may be involved by a load of tumor cells of advanced metastatic disease, causing increased extraction of radiopharmaceutical. The pattern should also be differentiated from other causes of diffusely increased uptake in the skeleton, or super scan, such as hyperparathyroidism, and other metabolic bone diseases which also show

Fig. 7.17 An example of cold metastatic lesions (*arrows*) in a patient with renal cell carcinoma of the right kidney which was surgically removed

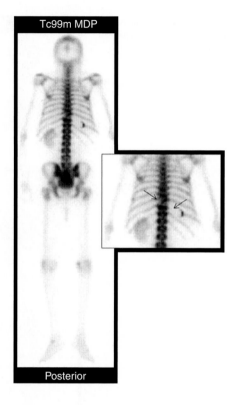

abnormal uptake extending to the skull, mandible, and variable length of long bones in addition to axial skeleton. Super scan secondary to metastases shows increased uptake that is usually confined to the axial skeleton (Fig. 7.18).

7.5
Summary

Nuclear Medicine today has an expanding role in the diagnosis of many bone diseases. Bone scintigraphy is one of the most common investigations performed in nuclear medicine and is used routinely in the evaluation of patients with cancer and in an expanding list of benign diseases. Since it is an extremely sensitive modality to evaluate a large spectrum of abnormalities related to the skeleton, it has been included for routine staging and restaging protocols for a variety of cancers which have a trend to develop bone metastases (e.g., breast, prostate, lung, and melanoma). In addition to the use in malignant disease its role in benign bone diseases has been expanding and is contributing to definite diagnosis of several skeletal conditions such as skeletal infection, radiologically occult fractures, complex regional pain syndrome, metabolic bone disease, and osteonecrosis. Recently, the 18 F-PET has added value to the role of nuclear medicine in bone diseases particularly malignant and enhanced the diagnostic impact of radionuclide bone studies.

Fig. 7.18 An example of diffuse metastatic disease. Note that the axial skeleton is predominantly involved

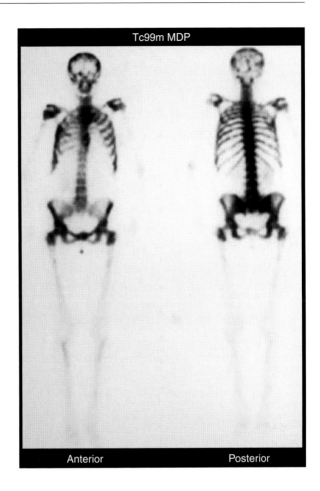

Tc99m MDP

Anterior   Posterior

Further Reading

Coleman RE (1997) Skeletal complications of malignancy. Cancer 80(suppl):1588–1594

Coleman RE (2001) Metastatic bone disease: clinical features, pathophysiology and treatment strategies. Cancer Treat Rev 27:165–176

Elgazzar A (2004) Orthopedic nuclear medicine. Springer, Berlin/New York

Evan-Sapir E (2005) Imaging of malignant bone involvement by morphologic, scintigraphic and hybrid modalities. J Nucl Med 46:1356–1367

Ferlay J, Bray F, Pisani P, Parkin DM, GLOBOCAN (2000) Cancer incidence, mortality and prevalence worldwide, version 1.0. IARC Cancer Base No. 5. IARC, Lyon. Available at: http://www-dep.iarc.fr/globocan/cdrom.htm

Palestro CJ, Love C (2007) Radionuclide imaging of musculoskeletal infection: convertional agents. Semin Musculoskeletal Radiol 11:335–352

Schauwecker DS (1992) The scintigraphic diagnosis of osteomyelitis. Am J Roentgenol 158:9–18

Cardiovascular System

8

Contents

8.1
Introduction

Nuclear medicine provides important information in the diagnosis and management of several cardiovascular disorders. It provides a noninvasive means for evaluation of cardiac function. Radionuclide imaging of myocardial perfusion is a commonly performed nuclear medicine examination to determine the adequacy of blood flow to the myocardium, especially in conjunction with exercise or pharmacologic stress for the detection and evaluation of coronary artery disease. Myocardial perfusion studies are obtained using one isotope commonly Tc99m compounds, dual isotope technique along with thalium-201,or more recently positron emission tomography which has added value in evaluation of myocardial metabolism for evaluation of myocardial viability. Nuclear medicine also helps in the diagnosis of hemangioma and lymphedema.

A.H. Elgazzar, *A Concise Guide to Nuclear Medicine*,
DOI: 10.1007/978-3-642-19426-9_8, © Springer-Verlag Berlin Heidelberg 2011

8.2
Clinical Uses

- Evaluation of cardiac function
- Evaluation of myocardial perfusion
- Evaluation of myocardial metabolism
- Diagnosis of soft tissue hemangioma
- Evaluation of lymph drainage

8.3
Evaluation of Cardiac Function

Noninvasive evaluation of cardiac function can be performed by continuous-loop imaging of the radiolabeled intracardiac blood pool such as Tc99m-labeled red blood cells. Regional wall motion as well as synchrony of contraction can be evaluated. The left ventricular ejection fraction (Normally ≥ 50%) and diastolic function can also be accurately measured. The cavity of the ventricle is visualized and evaluated by this study; however, the cardiac muscle is not itself seen. This *gated cardiac blood pool study* is used in the following clinical situations:

- Monitoring cardiotoxicity of chemotherapy such as doxorubicin
- Workup of heart failure
- Assessment of left and right ventricular volumes
- Prognosis after acute myocardial infarction
- Preoperative cardiac risk assessment

8.4
Evaluation of Myocardial Perfusion and Metabolism

Clinical manifestations of coronary artery disease include angina pectoris, myocardial infarction, congestive heart failure, and sudden death. It may be asymptomatic until advanced in severity. Most diagnostic methods, both invasive and noninvasive, depend on detection of luminal narrowing of the epicardial coronary vessels. Vessel narrowing of up to 75% of the cross-section area (or <50% of luminal narrowing) does not affect resting coronary flow. Increase of coronary flow caused by exercise or pharmacological stress exaggerates flow nonuniformity, through either increased metabolic demand or vasodilation. The easiest method of increasing coronary flow is physical exercise, using a motorized treadmill or a stationary bicycle. In patients who are unable to exercise adequately, pharmacological agents (adenosine, dipyridamole, dobutamine, and arbutamine) are used for transient elevation of coronary flow.

Myocardial perfusion imaging maps the relative distribution of coronary flow, which is normally almost uniform in the absence of prior infarction or fibrosis (Fig. 8.1). In the

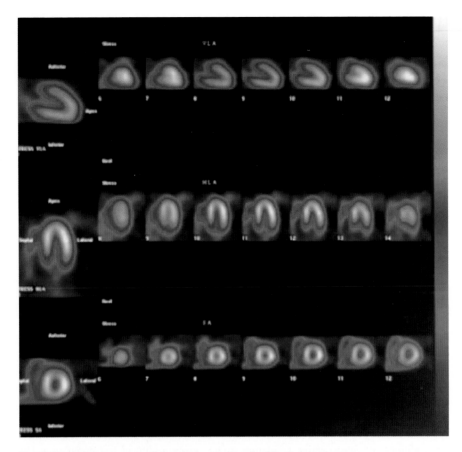

Fig. 8.1 Normal stress myocardial perfusion study using 99mTc myoview

presence of luminal narrowing, flow nonuniformity corresponds to anatomical location of the coronary stenosis and to the cumulative severity of the obstructions along the coronary arterial tree (Fig. 8.2). Therefore, myocardial perfusion imaging can diagnose not only the presence of coronary artery disease, but also its extent, severity, and physiological impact, thereby providing great prognostic power. The study is used in patients with or suspected of having CAD for:

- Diagnosis such as in acute chest syndrome, and diabetics to diagnose silent ischemia
- Prognosis
- Risk stratification in stable CAD
- Postacute myocardial infarction evaluation
- Evaluation after revascularization procedures
- Preoperative assessment
- Assessment of viability to detect hypoxic yet viable myocardium that would benefit from revascularization

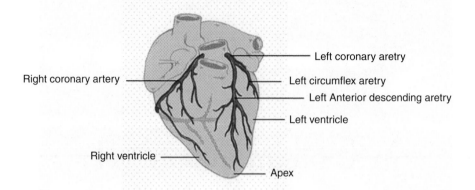

Right coronary artery

Left coronary aretry

Left circumflex aretry

Left Anterior descending aretry

Left ventricle

Right ventricle

Apex

Fig. 8.2 Diagram of the main structures of the heart and coronary arteries

8.4.1
Diagnosis

Average sensitivity and specificity of myocardial perfusion imaging for diagnosis of CAD have been reported close to 90% and 70%, respectively. The gold standard for diagnosis of CAD remains coronary angiography, despite its known limitations and likely systematic underestimation of the extent of disease. True sensitivity and specificity with each new tracer and each new imaging protocol has been difficult to ascertain because of post-test angiographic bias. Patients with negative results on MPI (Fig. 8.1) are rarely referred for coronary angiography. This practice is justified because of the known excellent prognosis of patients with a normal MPI study. Nevertheless, this limits the usefulness of retrospective validation studies using a clinical test population. On imaging ischemia appears as defect(s) on stress which improves or disappears on resting study (Figs. 8.3).

8.4.2
Prognosis

Myocardial perfusion imaging provides valuable risk stratification in stable CAD. Perfusion abnormalities can be classified according to size, localization, severity, and reversibility. Left ventricular volumes, systolic wall thickening, segmental wall motion, and ejection fraction can be quantified. Right ventricular size and function can be assessed.

A normal perfusion pattern in patients with an adequate level of stress and with high-quality study is consistent with an excellent short-term prognosis, regardless of coronary anatomy. Extent of perfusion abnormalities characterized by number of abnormal segments, severity of defects, and extent of reversibility (ischemia), define prognosis. When integrated with results of the exercise stress test and parameters of left and right ventricular

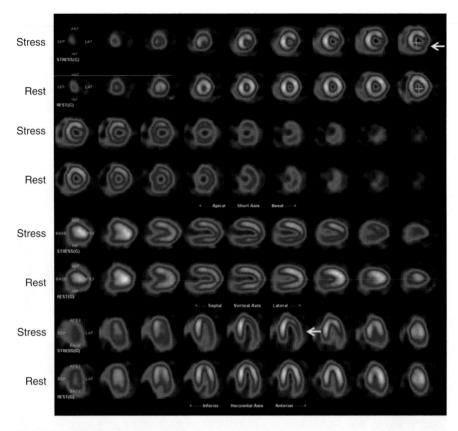

Fig. 8.3 Lateral wall ischemia (*arrows*)

function, combined information has a prognostic value which exceeds prognostication based on performance of coronary angiography. The average annual cardiac event rate in patients with abnormal images is 12-fold that in patients with normal images. Both fixed and reversible defects are prognostically significant. Fixed defects (Fig. 8.4) are a predictor of death, whereas reversible defects (Fig. 8.5) are an important predictor of nonfatal myocardial infarction. The event rate is significantly greater in patients with severe than in those with mild abnormalities.

8.4.3
Follow-Up After Acute Myocardial Infarction

The purposes of early or predischarge myocardial perfusion imaging evaluation after an acute myocardial infarction are (a) to assess the extent of sustained damage, including determination of the ejection fraction, and (b) to detect residual ischemia.

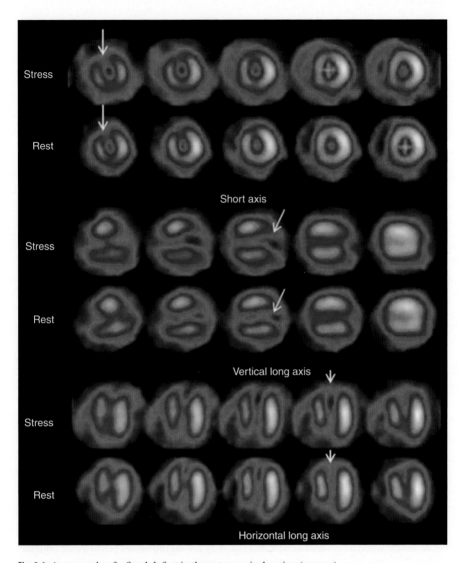

Fig. 8.4 An example of a fixed defect in the antero-apical region (*arrows*)

8.4.4
Follow-Up After Revascularization Procedures

In view of the possibility of restenosis after percutaneous revascularization and of coronary bypass graft closure after coronary artery bypass surgery, and the frequent absence of reliable symptoms, myocardial perfusion imaging is an efficient means to determine the need for additional and/or repeat interventions.

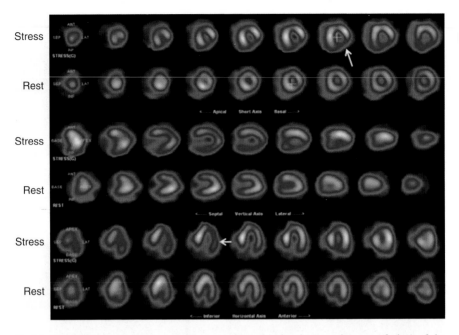

Fig. 8.5 Myocardial Perfusion Scan with stress-induced ischemia (complete reperfusion) of the inferolateral and anterior walls (*arrows*)

8.4.5
Preoperative Evaluation

This is particularly recommended for those patients with risk factors or signs or symptoms of coronary artery disease. The patient's risk factors include severity and/or stability of known heart disease, the presence of concomitant conditions such as diabetes mellitus, peripheral vascular disease, renal insufficiency, pulmonary disease, urgency of the surgery (emergency vs. elective), and type of surgery planned. Risk stratification based on preoperative testing can help the patient and physician choose the best type and timing of surgery, perioperative care, and long-term postoperative management.

8.4.6
Viability Assessment

Determining viability in patients with coronary artery disease is crucial to determine the proper course of management. Viability indicates justification of revascularization procedures. Although viability can be determined by thallium 201, it is best evaluated by F-18-FDG positron emission tomography (Figs. 8.6 and 8.7).

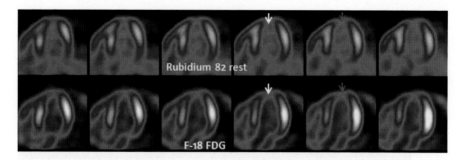

Fig. 8.6 Rubidium-82 Perfusion (*upper*) and metabolic (*lower*) images show no difference in an apical defect indicating a scar with no viability

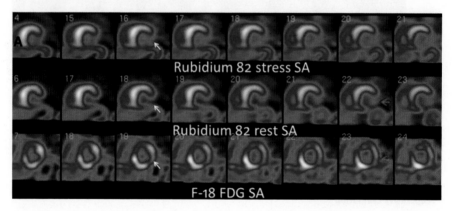

Fig. 8.7 Viable myocardium indicated by filling of the inferior–lateral defect by activity on FDG images (*arrows*) while is fixed on the perfusion study obtained utilizing Rubidium-82. *SA* = short axis

8.5
Soft Tissue Hemangioma Study

Soft tissue hemangiomas are the most common of the angiomatous lesions, representing around 7% of all benign soft tissue tumors in the general population with women being more affected. Depending on the predominant type of vascular channel, they are subdivided into five categories; capillary, cavernous, arteriovenous, venous, and mixed variations.

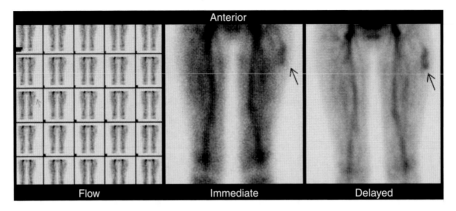

Fig. 8.8 Labeled red blood cell study of an 11-old-girl presented with diffuse antero–lateral swelling in upper one third of the thigh since birth. Dynamic perfusion images (**a**) show increased flow to left upper thigh region. Immediate (**b**) and delayed (**c**) spot views of the thighs in anterior and posterior projections show increased radiotracer activity in the upper one third of the thigh (*arrow*). Findings of soft tissue hemangioma

The technetium-labeled red blood cells scintigraphy helps to avoid unnecessary biopsy of the angiomatous lesions with the bleeding complications. The whole-body scanning using the Tc-labeled RBCs is helpful to determine the nature, multiplicity of lesions, and extent of the disease (Fig. 8.8).

8.6
Lymphoscintigraphy

Lymph is a body fluid with low protein content, high fat level, and circulating lymphocytes. Lymph drains from peripheral tissues in blind-ended lymph vessels passing through lymph nodes and ending into the central venous circulation. Failure of lymph drainage from an area of the body results in lymphedema. Lymph drainage can be studied by following the movement of radiolabeled microparticles injected intradermally by scintillation camera imaging (Fig. 8.9). The study is used in:

- Primary and secondary lymphedema due to surgery or irradiation
- Progressing edema without an obvious etiology

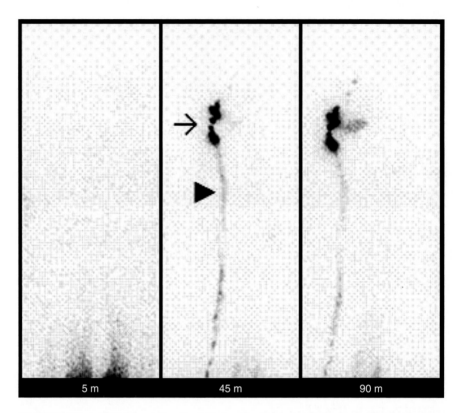

Fig. 8.9 Lymphoscintigraphy study of a patient with right lower limb edema. The 5 min image shows beginning of ascent of the radiotracer from the injection sites. The 45 and 90 min images shown illustrates normal drainage of the radionuclide in the left side with visualization of inguinal lymph nodes (*arrow*) and lymph channels (*arrow head*) and lack of migration in the right side due to obstruction

8.7
Summary

Nuclear medicine is an important component in the diagnosis and management of heart disease. Cardiac angiography provides excellent images of the anatomy coronary arteries. On the other hand nuclear medicine studies provide additional information by showing the regional perfusion and function of the myocardium. It also provides prognostic information in patients known to have coronary artery disease. Nuclear medicine also helps in accurate diagnosis of soft tissue hemangiomas and lymphedema of the upper and lower extremities.

Further Reading

Delbeke D, Vitola JV (2004) Nuclear cardiology and correlative imaging. Springer, Berlin

Douglas Miller D (2009) Cost effeciency of Nuclear cardiology services in the mordern health care environment. Journal of Nuclear Cardiology 16:41–52

Heiba S, Zubaid M (2006) Basis of cardiac imaging 1: myocardial contractility and assessment of cardiac function. In: Elgazzar AH (ed) Pathophysiologic basis of nuclear medicine, 2nd edn. Springer, Berlin, pp 305–329

Machac J (2006) Basis of cardiac imaging 2: myocardial perfusion, metabolism, infarction and receptor imaging in coronary artery disease and congestive heart failure. In: Elgazzar A, Elgazzar AH (eds) Pathophysiologic basis of nuclear medicine, 2nd edn. Springer, Berlin, pp 330–351

Nawaz K, Hamad MM, Sadek S, Awdeh M, Eklof B, Abdel-Dayem HM (1986) Dynamic lymph flow imaging in lymphedema: normal and abnormal patterns. Clin Nucl Med 11:653–658

Vitola JV, Shaw LJ, Allam AH, Orellana P, Peix A, et al. (2009) Assessing the need for Nuclear cardiology and other advanced cardiac imaging. Journal of Nuclear Cardiology 16:956–961

Central Nervous System

9

Contents

9.1
Introduction

Cerebral blood flow and metabolism are generally interconnected. Alterations in brain function are associated with corresponding changes in perfusion. Radionuclide brain perfusion studies using lipophilic tracers are useful in the study of abnormalities of regional perfusion such as stroke and in the evaluation of changes related to neuronal activity like epilepsy and trauma. Their use in psychiatric conditions is promising. Several radiopharmaceuticals are used for imaging central nervous system. These include 99mTc HMPAO (Fig. 9.1), F-18 FDG (Fig. 9.2), and less commonly In111 DTPA.

A.H. Elgazzar, *A Concise Guide to Nuclear Medicine*,
DOI: 10.1007/978-3-642-19426-9_9, © Springer-Verlag Berlin Heidelberg 2011

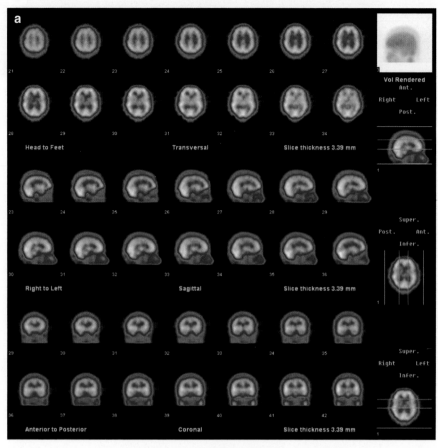

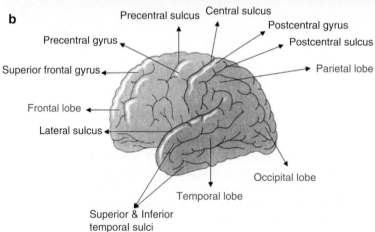

Fig. 9.1 Normal brain perfusion study using 99mTc-HMPAO showing adequate and uniform activity in different areas (**a**) corresponding to the normal structures of the brain as seen in the diagram (**b**)

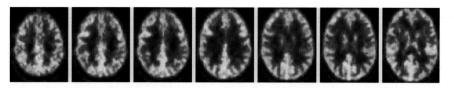

Fig. 9.2 Normal brain FDG-PET

9.2
Clinical Uses

- Dementia especially Alzheimer's disease and AIDS dementia
- Partial complex epilepsy and localization of seizure foci
- Cerebrovascular insufficiency: Location, size, and prognosis of cerebral ischemia and stroke
- Diagnosis of brain death
- Brain injury
- Recurrent brain tumors after surgery and irradiation
- Diagnosis and follow-up of certain cerebrospinal fluid disorders

9.3
Dementia

Dementia can be broadly categorized as resulting from vascular disease or from a progressive degenerative process. Brain SPECT imaging using regional cerebral blood flow (rCBF) tracers is useful to distinguish these two classes of dementia.

Alzheimer's disease (the most common progressive degenerative dementia) is characterized by low global blood flow with accentuation of the diminution in the posterior temporal parietal lobes (Fig. 9.3), relative sparing of the thalamus and corpus striatum, as well as the somatomotor sensory cortex, and late involvement of the frontal lobes.

9.4
Brain Death

Death is an irreversible, biological event that consists of permanent cessation of the critical functions of the organism as a whole. It implies permanent absence of cerebral and brainstem functions. It then qualifies as death (as brain is essential for integrating critical functions of the body). The equivalence of brain death with death is largely but not universally accepted.

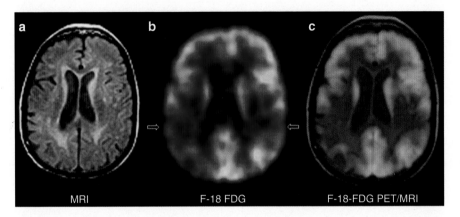

Fig. 9.3 FDG-PET study of Alzheimer's disease. MRI scan (**a**) reveals chronic small vessel ischemic changes and mild diffuse atrophy without a specific pattern which would be diagnostic for Alzheimer's disease. F-18 FDG brain PET scan (**b**) shows activity reduction involving the posterior temporal and parietal lobes bilaterally, right more severely affected as compared to the left. F-18 FDG brain PET scan fused with the T1-weighted MRI scan (**c**) shows in the areas of decreased F-18 FDG uptake there is no cerebral atrophy out of proportion with other areas of the brain to indicate that the reduction of F-18 FDG uptake is an atrophy effect, and therefore decreased F-18 FDG uptake can be attributed to reduced neuronal metabolic activity as a result of neuronal impairment attributable to the amyloidopathy of Alzheimer's disease

The concept of irreversible coma or brain death was first described in 1959, predating widespread organ donation. The fundamental definition of brain death has substantively remained constant over time and across countries (although specific details of diagnostic criteria differ). Many conditions are known to cause brain death (Table 9.1).

Diagnosis of brain death is clinical with tests available for confirmation and documentation. These confirmatory tests include:

1. EEG with no physiologic brain activity
2. Absent cerebral circulation on angiography or scintigraphy (the principal legal sign in USA and many European countries)
3. Confirmatory imaging for brain death:

   (a) Cerebral angiography
       Lack of intracranial perfusion other than filling of the superior sagittal sinus is strongly confirmatory of brain death on a selective 4-vessel angiogram with iodinated contrast medium.
   (b) Radionuclide scanning

Table 9.1 Causes of brain death

Trauma and subarachnoid hemorrhage (most common)
Intracerebral hemorrhage
Hypoxic ischemic encephalopathy
Ischemic stroke
Any condition causing permanent widespread brain injury

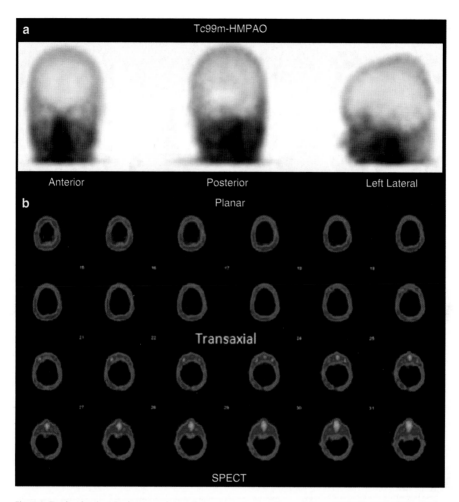

Fig. 9.4 Brain death: No intracranial activity is seen on planar (**a**) or SPECT (**b**). Compare to Fig. 9.1 where activity is present indicating no brain death

No tracer uptake in the brain parenchyma indicates brain death (Fig. 9.4). This study is increasingly used as an alternative to cerebral angiography. Imaging is done using a radioactively labeled substance that readily crosses the blood–brain barrier such as 99mTc-HMPAO.

9.5
Seizure Localization

Epilepsy is a disorder in which repeated episodes of seizures occur with or without an identifiable primary brain disease. Epilepsy affects about 0.5% of the population and usually begins in childhood, but it can affect people at any age. Seizures result when a focus

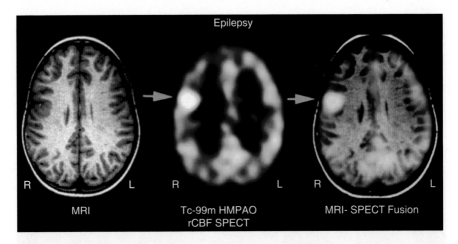

Fig. 9.5 Frontal lobe epilepsy in a 9-year-old right-handed boy. The MRI scan (*left*) is normal. 99mTc-HMPAO study (*middle*) shows a focus of increased uptake (*arrow*) reflecting the regional cerebral perfusion at the time the tracer was injected during the epileptogenic seizure. The abnormality is better localized on the fused image with MRI study (*right*)

of neuronal discharge is propagated indiscriminately within the brain by an abnormal neuronal electrochemical process. This process can be detected as electrical activity by an electroencephalograph (EEG).

The use of Tc-99m-HMPAO in epilepsy patient during the ictal state (Fig. 9.5) or PET FDG during interictal phase is valuable in localizing detecting and epileptic foci in difficult cases where other modalities cannot provide accurate localization.

9.6
Brain Tumor

The current therapy of malignant high-grade tumor is suboptimal, partly because of the difficulty in distinguishing recurrent viable tumor from cerebral necrosis resulting from effective therapy or radiation therapy. Conventional CT or MRI shows mass effect, edema, and contrast enhancement in both cases. Metabolic imaging can assist to differentiate these processes since effective therapy results in decreased tumor growth and metabolism, while suboptimal treatment will result in tumor regrowth and increased uptake of radionuclide markers of metabolism (Fig. 9.6). PET has been successful in differentiating post-therapy changes from tumor recurrence (Fig. 9.7). Additionally it has also been successful in determining the prognosis as it can more accurately predict the degree of malignancy than CT and MRI.

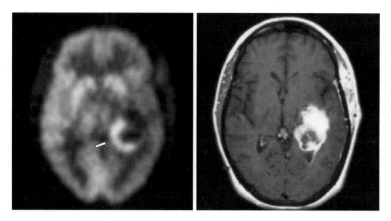

Fig. 9.6 A 47-year-old with left temporal lobe tumor. F-18-FDG PET study (*left*) obtained 1 month after surgical resection shows residual high-grade tumor (*arrow*) which is not clear within the significant postsurgical changes seen on MRI (*right*)

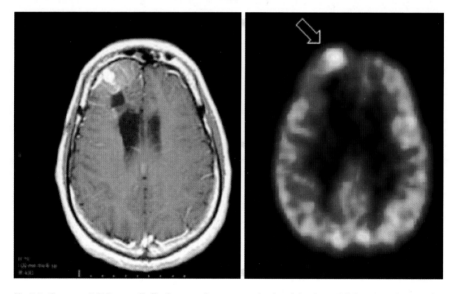

Fig. 9.7 Contrast MRI scan (*left*) shows enhancement in the right frontal lobe. F-18 FDG_PET study (*right*) shows a focal area of increased F-18 FDG uptake (*arrow*) involving the right frontal lobe consistent with high-grade transformation and recurrence of tumor in the right frontal lobe 8 years after initial diagnosis, therapy, and complete remission

9.7
Cerebrospinal Fluid Abnormalities

The cerebrospinal fluid (CSF), with a total volume of 150 mL, provides a mechanical buffer to the central nervous system. It is produced by the choriod plexus at a rate of 500 mL per day. The CSF drains into the sagittal sinus through absorption by the arachnoid villi and Pacchioni granules. Mechanical obstruction of the brain ventricular system or absorption failure of the CSF at the granules leads to dilatation of the ventricular system called hydrocephalus with associated clinical disturbances. These abnormalities can be studied by introducing radiotracers intrathecally via a lumbar puncture and following their fate by scintillation imaging (Radionuclide Cisternoscintigraphy). This study is used to diagnose:

- Normal pressure hydrocephalus
- Hydrocephalus due to obstruction of the ventricular and duct system
- Cerebrospinal fluid leak (rhinorrhea or otorrhea)
- Evaluation of ventricular shunt patency

Abnormalities of CSF drainage can be corrected by the placement of artificial shunting from the lateral ventricle to the peritoneal cavity. Other similar devices are used for drug delivery in CNS tumors. Radionuclide shunt studies are valuable also in monitoring the patency of these devices.

9.8
Summary

Nuclear medicine has in general a limited role in the central nervous system disorders. CT and MRI have a more important role in imaging CNS. In certain conditions nuclear medicine can provide more reliable information that cannot be obtained from other imaging modalities. It is important in early diagnosis of Alzheimer disease and the differential diagnosis of dementia. It provides a crucial help in confirming brain death, evaluation of brain tumor recurrence, and in the evaluation and follow-up of certain cerebrospinal fluid disorders. Preoperative localization of seizure foci can also be achieved in difficult cases by nuclear medicine imaging.

Further Reading

Gary R, Sinha P (2003) Scintigraphy as a confirmatory test of brain death. Semin Nucl Med 33:312
Ishibashi K, Saito Y, Murayama S, Kanemaru K, Oda K, Ishiwata K, Mizusawa H, Ishii K (2010) Validation of cardiac I-123 MIBG scintigraphy in patients with Parkinson disease who were diagnosed with dopa-mine PET. Eur J Nucl Med Mol Imaging 37:3–11
Mountz JM, San Pedro EC (2006) Basis and clinical application of functional brain imaging. In: Elgazzar AH (ed) Pathophysiologic basis of nuclear medicine, 2nd edn. Springer, Berlin

Nuclear Oncology

10

Contents

10.1
Introduction

Nuclear medicine has a major role in the management of malignant tumors. With the developments toward molecular imaging and the advancement of equipment used for imaging particularly after combining the nuclear medicine instruments with morphologic modalities, it has even become a more integral part of management protocols. This role includes detection of malignant tumors, staging and restaging of the disease, early detection of recurrence, evaluation of the response to therapy, and prediction of the prognosis. Additionally sentinel node identification and localization for biopsy is another important use of nuclear medicine to help plan the most suitable management for several tumors. The main tumor imaging radiopharmaceutical can be summarized as shown in Table 10.1.

A.H. Elgazzar, *A Concise Guide to Nuclear Medicine*,
DOI: 10.1007/978-3-642-19426-9_10, © Springer-Verlag Berlin Heidelberg 2011

Table 10.1 Main Tumor imaging radiopharmaceuticals

Nonspecific agents
Ga-67
Tl-201
Tc99m-Sestamibi
Tc99m MDP
Fluorine-18-FDG
Specific agents
I-131/I-123
In-111/Tc99m Octreotide
Monoclonal antibodies
I-131/I-123 MIBG

10.2
Clinical Uses

- Diagnosis of Tumors
- Pretreatment staging of malignant disease
- Detection of residual or recurrent disease
- Evaluating response to therapy
- Radiotherapy planning
- Sentinel lymph node localization

10.3
Diagnosis of Tumors

Generally, nuclear medicine has limited role in primary tumor detection, however it helps in the detection and characterization of certain tumors. Examples include evaluation of nodular thyroid disease as nodules that may be malignant (see Chap. 3). Scinti-mamography is another example used in selected patients when mammography is not conclusive. It is a simple procedure using intravenous injection of Tc99m MIBI followed by early and delayed imaging of the breasts and can indicate the nature of visualized lesions (Figs. 10.1 and 10.2). Positron emission mamography (PEM) is recent being used in such cases. PET/CT is also increasingly used for managing many types of cancer including detection. Evaluation of the nature of solitary lung nodule (Fig. 10.3) and, in certain cases, of suspected breast cancer (Fig. 10.4) and tumor detection in cases with unknown primary are examples.

10.4
Staging of Malignant Disease

Staging of cancer depends on the size of the primary neoplasm, its extent to regional lymph nodes, and the presence or absence of metastasis. Accurate staging of malignant lesions at the time of initial presentation is of utmost importance to provide appropriate

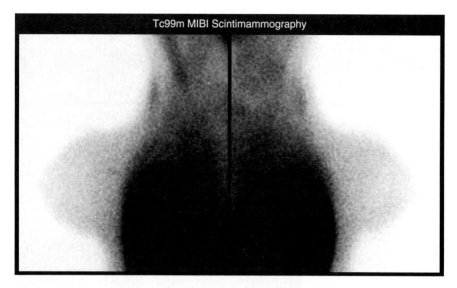

Fig. 10.1 Negative radionuclide mammography study

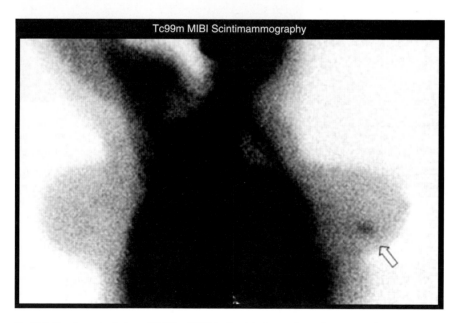

Fig. 10.2 Focal accumulation of Tc99m MIBI in the right breast (*arrow*) proven to be cancer

management for a particular patient. Overstaging can inappropriately deprive a patient from receiving curative treatment such as surgery. On the other hand understaging can subject a patient to undergo futile but drastic treatments that can even increase the morbidity and mortality (e.g., pneumonectomy in lung cancer) without any increase in the chance of cure (see also Chap. 6).

Fig. 10.3 Solitary lung nodule
with high FDG activity
(*arrow*) indicating malignancy that was proven later

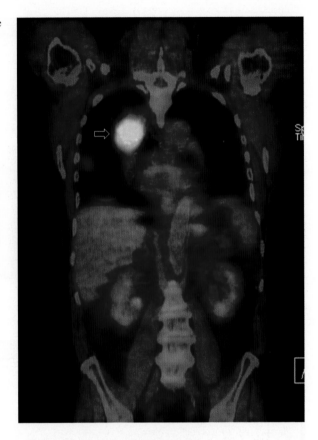

Imaging plays a significant role in staging. Bone imaging using Tc99m MDP and
F-18 has established value in detecting metastatic bone disease (see Chap. 7). Similarly,
several radiopharmaceuticals are used in staging and follow-up of neuroendocrine
tumors (see Chap. 4).

Although the ideal staging is a microscopic process, many times it is not possible to
biopsy each and every lesion to find out whether they are malignant or not. Nuclear medicine procedures, especially F-18 FDG-PET, have a higher degree of accuracy compared
with CT or MRI alone in staging tumors particularly lymph node involvement.

CT criteria for staging lymph node involvement depend mostly on the size of the lymph
nodes. If they are more than 1 cm in the mediastinum for example, the lymph nodes are
considered to be positive for malignant involvement. However, microscopic involvement
of these lymph nodes is not related to their size. Metastatic malignant cells can involve
small lymph nodes on the other hand, large lymph nodes can be due to inflammatory
response without metastatic involvement. MRI has the advantage of functionally verifying
and determining whether the draining lymph nodes are involved by metastatic invasion.
The accuracy of CT in staging mediastinal disease in lung cancer as an example is approximately 70%; MRI is slightly higher at around 80%, while F-18 FDG accuracy is better
than 90%.

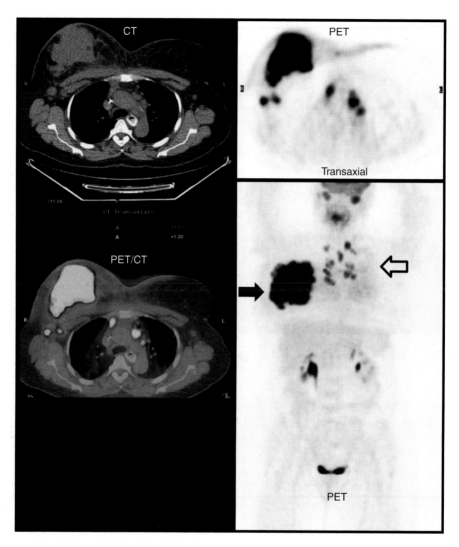

Fig. 10.4 F-18 FDG-PET/CT study showing primary tumor in the right breast (*solid arrow*) and foci of lymph node involvement (*open arrow*)

10.5
Detection of Residual or Recurrent Disease

The role of identifying viable tumors by imaging is increasing because of the problems encountered by MRI and CT, especially after surgical, radiation, or chemotherapy treatment in differentiating post-therapy changes from residual viable tumor tissue, local recurrence, or necrosis. As a result different radiopharmaceuticals play an important role

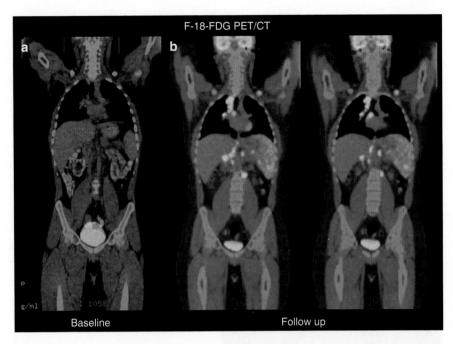

Fig. 10.5 Baseline (**a**) and follow-up (**b**) F-18-FDG-PET/CT studies of a 21-year-old man with Hodgkin's lymphoma. The follow-up shows recurrent tumor at multiple lymph nodes and spleen

in different malignancies and for detecting recurrence (Fig. 10.5). PET, and if not available, thaliun-201, helps in detecting tumor recurrence and in differentiating tumor recurrence from necrosis as post-therapy changes that is difficult to differentiate based on CT or MRI.

10.6
Evaluating Response to Therapy

Patients can respond differently to the same treatment protocol and accordingly individualization of therapy should be more appropriate. However, as tumors and their hosts are heterogeneous, there are many crucial secondary problems related to the individualization of therapy. The most important element in individualization of therapy is to be able to rapidly assess whether a chosen treatment strategy is effective. Tumor volume changes observed during follow-up CT or MRI studies in principle can be used for evaluation of response to antitumor therapy. However, it is not early enough before the patient develops considerable toxicity and side effects from the prescribed chemotherapy.

Radiopharmaceutical agents like Gallium in lymphoma (Fig. 10.6) and FDG in many tumors such as Lymphoma, lung, head and neck cancer, breast cancer and others (Figs. 10.7–10.8) have shown good results to predict response to a treatment regimen as early as after 1–3 cycles of chemotherapy.

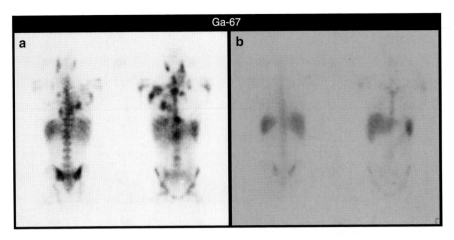

Fig. 10.6 Ga-67 study (**a**) in a patient with non-Hodgkin's lymphoma. Follow-up study (**b**) shows clearly an excellent response to chemotherapy evidenced by clearing of the foci of uptake noted in the first pretherapy study

10.7
Radiotherapy Planning

CT has a high diagnostic ability by visualizing lesion morphology and by providing the exact localization of sites but lacks the information of the functional status. Whereas, Positron Emission Tomography (PET) with fluorine-18 fluorodeoxyglucose (FDG) provides information about the metabolism and viability of the lesions but fails to provide precise topographic localization.

Fused images from FDG-PET and CT provides valuable information resulting in more accurate delineation of normal tissues from tumor-bearing areas at high risk for recurrence compared with CT alone and PET/CT can improve the therapeutic window for radiation therapy. Image fusion is also reported to increase the confidence of the radiation oncologist while drawing target volumes and thereby, reduces the interobserver variation.

10.8
Sentinel Lymph Node Localization

This is relatively a recent trend for identifying the sentinel node(s) which represents the first drain for the primary tumor and is particularly used in breast Cancer, Cutaneous Melanoma, Squamous Cell Carcinoma of Head and Neck, and colorectal cancer. Tracer (Tc99m radiolabeled particles) is injected into a specific location based on tumor type, and they are retained in the lymph nodes because of their localization within RES cells. Radioactive sentinel nodes can be detected using imaging with a gamma camera and/or a gamma probe at surgery.

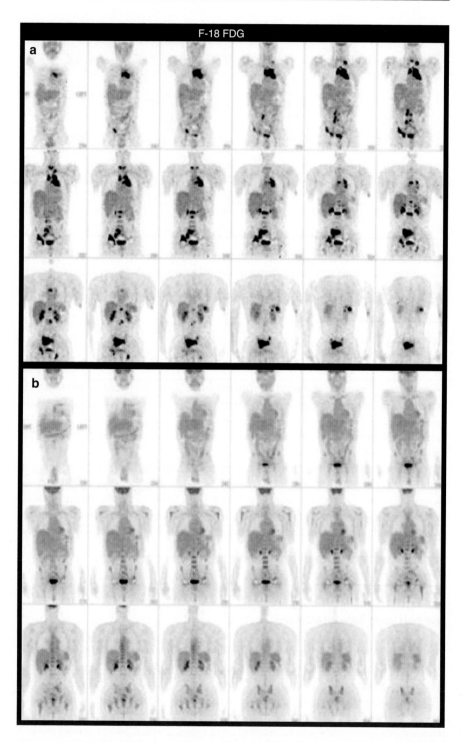

Fig. 10.7 (a) FDG-PET pretherapy study of a patient with nonHodgkin's lymphoma (b) Follow-up study showing favorable response to therapy with clearing of the uptake in multiple foci in the chest and abdomen

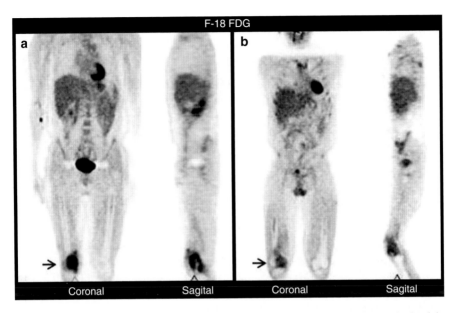

Fig. 10.8 Initial (**a**) and follow-up (**b**) F-18 FDG of a patient with osteogenic sarcoma in the right distal femur (*arrow*) showing decreasing uptake in the follow-up study after chemotherapy indicating favorable response to therapy

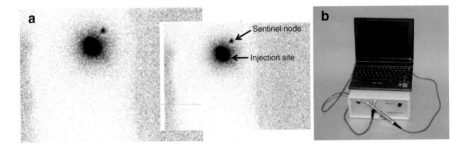

Fig. 10.9 (**a**) Sentinel node visualization (*arrow*) in a patient with breast cancer. (**b**) an example of a gamma probe which is used during surgery for localization with no need for imaging

Although sentinel node imaging does not image the cancer, it can identify the lymph node/nodes where the primary tumor drains. Excision followed by immunohistological staining of the sentinel node can identify micrometastases. At the present time, sentinel lymph node localization technique is the most acceptable alternative to routine total node dissection (Fig. 10.9) such as axillary dissection in breast cancer.

10.9
Summary

Proper Management of Cancer requires evaluation of tumor extent, monitoring of therapy, and evaluation of treatment-induced side effects. Imaging modalities are crucial in achieving all the three main prerequisites for the proper management. Structural modalities such as CT and functional modalities such as gamma camera imaging are complementary rather than competitive for cancer management. Each modality has advantages and limitations. Positron emission tomography (PET) as a recent functional modality is now the most powerful modality in advancing cancer management. F-18 FDG PET is a noninvasive, 3-dimensional imaging modality that has become widely used in the management of patients with cancer.

Due to lack of anatomical details nuclear medicine tracers are not preferred for T-staging which will change in the era of PET/CT when we have both functional and anatomical information needed for T staging; however, due to superior ability to detect lymph node (N) and distant metastases (M), nuclear medicine techniques particularly FDG-PET plays a significant role for N & M staging of several cancers such as lung, head and neck, esophagus, colorectal, lymphoma, and melanoma.

Individual tumors will vary widely in their response to a particular form of therapy. Early, particularly after 1–3 cycles of chemotherapy, identification of tumors that are not responding to conventional therapies would permit the timely institution of alternative treatment that may be more effective. FDG-PET imaging can evaluate tumor response to therapy before anatomic changes are observed. PET imaging is currently the most sensitive and specific imaging method to obtain information about tumor physiology. FDG-PET imaging can have significant impact on clinical treatment decisions by providing a more timely and accurate assessment of treatment efficacy. Assessment of tumor response to therapy can be determined by visual assessment of the images or by quantitative analysis using standard uptake values.

Further Reading

Bahl S, Alavi A, Basu S, Czerniecki BJ (2009) The role of PET and PET/CT in the surgical management of breast cancer: a review. PET Clin 4:277–287

Eubank WB, Lee JH, Mankoff DA (2009) Disease restaging and diagnosis of recurrent and metastatic disease following primary therapy with FDG-PET imaging. PET Clin 4:299–312

Francis IR, Brown RKJ, Avram AM (2005) The clinical role of CT/PET in oncology: an update. Cancer Imaging 5:S68–S75

Jana S, Abdel-Dayem HM (2006) Basis of tumor imaging; scintigraphic and pathophysiologic correlation. In: Elgazzar AH (ed) Pathophysiologic basis of nuclear medicine, 2nd edn. Springer, Berlin-New York

Roses RE, Kumar R, Alavi A, Czerniecki BJ (2009) The role of lymphatic mapping and sentinel lymph node biopsy in the staging of breast cancer. PET Clin 4:265–276

Tateishi U, Yamaguchi U, Seki K, Terauchi T, Arai Y, Hasegawa T (2006) Glut-1 expression and enhanced glucose metabolism are associated with tumor grade in bone and soft tissue. Eur J Nucl Med Mol Imaging 33:683–691

Therapeutic Applications of Nuclear Medicine

11

Contents

11.1
Introduction

Therapeutic applications of nuclear medicine are expanding (Table 11.1). The radioiso-topes in therapy were limited predominantly to treatment of hyperthyroidism and thyroid cancer, and polycythemia rubra vera for many years. Strontium 89 (Sr-89), rhenium 186 (Re-186), samarium 153 (Sm-153), and tin 117 m (Sn-117) have been increasingly used recently in treating bone pain secondary to metastases. Additionally, treatment of certain neuroendocrine tumors with I-131 MIBG and labeled octreotide and pentreotide, the use of radiolabeled monoclonal antibodies for lymphomas, and radionuclide synovectomy has revolutionized the field of therapeutic nuclear medicine.

A.H. Elgazzar, *A Concise Guide to Nuclear Medicine*,
DOI: 10.1007/978-3-642-19426-9_11, © Springer-Verlag Berlin Heidelberg 2011

Table 11.1 Therapeutic applications of Nuclear Medicine

Oncologic

Lymphomas and leukemia

Polycythemia rubra vera

Solid tumors (thyroid carcinoma, neuroblastoma, ovarian, prostate, breast, osteogenic sarcoma, others)

Treatment of metastasis-induced bone pain

Treatment of hepatic tumors

Nononcologic

Benign thyroid disease particularly hyperthyroidism

Radionuclide synovectomy

Bone marrow ablation

Intravascular radionuclide therapy for prevention of restenosis.

Generally, treatment options for cancer may be local (surgery or external beam radiation) or systemic. The role of nuclear medicine focuses on a targeted systemic approach, whether dealing with a primary tumor or with its metastatic foci.

11.2
Clinical Uses

- Treatment of hyperthyroidism and other benign thyroid conditions
- Treatment of differentiated thyroid cancer
- Treatment of pain secondary to skeletal metastases
- Treatment of neuroendocrine tumors
- Radioimmunotherapy
- Radionuclide synovectomy
- Peptide receptor radionuclide therapy

11.3
Treatment of Hyperthyroidism and Other Benign Thyroid Conditions

For more than 60 years, iodine-131 has been used to treat most cases of Graves' disease and hyperfunctioning nodules. It has become the modality of choice in treating Graves' disease, with the result that surgeons are becoming less and less experienced in thyroidectomy since the number of operations has decreased significantly. The normal thyroid gland utilizes iodine for the synthesis of thyroid hormones. The cells of the gland do not differentiate between stable iodine and radioactive iodine. Accordingly, if radioactive iodine is administered, it is trapped and then organified by thyroid follicular cells exactly like nonradioactive iodine.

After oral administration, I-131 iodide is absorbed rapidly from the upper gastrointestinal tract, 90% within 60 min. After entering the blood stream, the iodide is distributed in the extrathyroid compartment similar to the stable iodide and leaves this compartment to be taken up by the thyroid and by renal excretion. Approximately 20% of the administered activity is taken up normally by the thyroid gland. A small amount of I-131 is also found in the salivary glands, gastric mucosa, choroid plexus, breast milk, and placenta. Up to 75% is excreted by the kidney and 10% by fecal excretion.

The therapeutic effects of I-131 sodium iodide are due to the emission of ionizing radiation from the decaying radionuclide. In benign conditions such as Graves' disease, division of some metabolically active cells is prevented by the effect of this ionizing radiation. Cell death is another mechanism activated when the cells are exposed to high levels of radiation, particularly when high doses are given to patients with toxic adenoma, where the suppressed normal thyroid tissue is essentially spared with delivery of a very high concentration to the cells of the toxic nodule. Cell death is followed by replacement with connective tissue, which may lead to hypothyroidism, depending on the number of cells destroyed and replaced by fibrous nonfunctioning tissue. Since 90% of the radiation effects of I-131 are due to beta radiation, which has a short range in tissue of 0.5 mm, the extrathyroid radiations, and consequently the side effects, are minimal.

11.4
Treatment of Differentiated Thyroid Cancer

Radioactive iodine is the mainstay of therapy for residual, recurrent, and metastatic thyroid cancer that takes up iodine and cannot be resected.

About 90% or more of thyroid carcinomas are well differentiated, of the papillary, papillofollicular, follicular, and Hürthle-cell types, which take up iodine and accordingly can be successfully treated with I-131. The therapeutic effects on differentiated thyroid cancer, where larger doses of radioactive iodide are administered, is based on destruction of cells of the residual thyroid tissue and the functioning carcinoma cells by the high dose of administered radionuclide.

The mortality of patients treated with less than total thyroidectomy and limited I-131 therapy was found to be three to four times higher than that of patients treated with total thyroidectomy and adequate ADI-131 therapy to ablate known foci of radioiodine uptake.

11.5
Treatment of Pain Secondary to Skeletal Metastases

Approximately 75% of patients with advanced cancer have pain, with a high percentage due to skeletal metastases. Bone metastases cause intractable pain, which affects the quality of life for the patient, especially if it is associated with immobility, anorexia, and anxiety, with the consequent long-term use of narcotic analgesics. The mechanism of bone pain may not be clear in many of these patients and could be due to cell-secreted pain modulators such as interleukin-1 beta, interleukin-8, and interferon. Depending on the extent of bone metastases, radiation therapy or radiopharmaceuticals can be used instead of narcotics to alleviate the pain with the objective of improving the quality of life.

Bone-seeking radiopharmaceuticals emitting beta particles have been used to deliver local radiotherapy to metastases to decrease pain at their sites. Radiopharmaceuticals which are taken up at the sites of bone metastases will cause less toxicity than external radiation therapy. These radiopharmaceuticals control pain while causing only transient bone marrow depression, which is usually mild. The uptake of these radiopharmaceuticals by metastases is several-fold (up to 15–20 times) that of normal bone. These agents are absorbed to hydroxyapatite crystals at the site of active new bone, similar to Tc99m-MDP. They include phosphorus-32, strontium 89, rhenium 186 diphosphonate, and samarium-153 EDTMP. The list of radiopharmaceuticals for bone palliation has been increasing including Re-188, Lu-177 and others.

Radiopharmaceutical therapy is indicated for the treatment of patients with painful widespread bone metastases.

The response to these radiopharmaceuticals is more or less similar, with an average success rate of 70–80%.

11.6
Treatment of Neuroendocrine Tumors

Several neuroendocrine tumors are candidates for radionuclide therapy. The goals of radionuclide therapy for neuroendocrine tumors are to control symptom and pain to improve the quality of life, reduce medical requirements, and stabilize the disease, additionally, in limited disease to reduce tumor volume, reduce hormone secretion, and complete remission.

I-131 meta iodobenzylguanidine (MIBG) is being used in increasing trials and applications for therapy. It is used for the treatment of pheochromocytoma, malignant paraganglioma, neuroblastoma, medullary thyroid carcinoma, and symptomatic carcinoid tumors. The radiopharmaceutical resembles guanethidine and is concentrated by normal and abnormal sympathetic adrenergic tissue.

When I-131 MIBG is administered intravenously, it is transported by blood to be taken up by normal adrenergic tissue such as the adrenal medulla and sympathetic nervous system and by tumors of neuroectoderm-derived tissue. The uptake by these tumors is secondary to active neuronal uptake-1 mechanism and passive diffusion through the cell membrane, followed by active intracellular transport to the neurosecretory granules in the cytoplasm, where it is retained.

In normal adrenergic tissue such as the adrenal medulla, heart, and salivary glands, as well as in pheochromocytoma, 90% of MIBG is stored in the neurosecretory granules, while in neuroblastoma it was found that up to 60% is stored within the extragranular cells. The major part of the radiopharmaceutical is excreted unchanged in urine. The radiation effect is due to emission of beta particles from the decaying I-131 with a mechanism similar to that in treating thyroid disorders.

11.7
Radioimmunotherapy

Monoclonal antibodies are now contributing increasingly to cancer treatment, Y-90 and I-131 anti-CD-20 and I-131 anti-CD-22 are good examples which are used for non-Hodgkin's lymphomas. These antibodies can be used alone to kill tumor cells or conjugated with drugs, cytotoxic agents, and radionuclides to improve their effects.

Radioimmunotherapy using monoclonal antibodies conjugated with isotopes allows the delivery of radiation to tumor tissue while sparing normal tissue. This radiation can be administered as a single large dose of radiolabeled monoclonal antibodies or, more commonly, in multiple fractions.

The use of radioimmunotherapy for treating lymphoma has been expanding in the last decade. It is currently being used for recurrent and relapsed disease of low-grade B-cell, follicular, and transformed lymphomas.

11.8
Radionuclide Synovectomy

There may be a need for a definitive solution to the joint pain of many arthropathies, particularly rheumatoid arthritis, after failure of conventional medications. Therapeutic nuclear medicine offers an alternative to surgical synovectomy. Several radiopharmaceuticals can destroy the synovial membrane when injected intraarticularly (radionuclide synovectomy or radiosynoviorthesis) and the patients become pain free.

11.8.1
Radiopharmaceuticals for Synovectomy

Ytterium-90 colloid, erbium 169 citrate colloid, rhenium-186 colloid, Phosphorus-32 (P-32) colloid, and others are all used to treat synovial disease. Since these colloids vary in their physical characteristics and thus in their range of penetrability, they are used differently to achieve the therapeutic effects and avoid injuring the surrounding tissue. Accordingly, some radiopharmaceuticals are used for the knee while others are used for small joints. Yttrium-90 citrate or silicate is generally used for big joints such as the knee, rhenium-186 colloid is used for the shoulder, elbow, hip, and ankle, and erbium-169 citrate for the small joints in the hands and feet.

11.8.2
Clinical Use

Hemophiliac patients with chronic synovitis and hemarthropathy, rheum atoid arthritis, pigmented villonodular synovitis, psoriatic arthritis, ankylosing spondylitis, and collagenosis are candidates for this treatment modality. Furthermore, persistent effusion after joint prosthesis is a relative indication.

Two or three-phase bone scan should be obtained before planning therapy to assess the degree of inflammation of the joint and soft tissue and in order to be able to decide if radiosynovectomy is possible and if the patient would benefit from this therapy. Scintigraphy is particularly important to evaluate the extent of abnormalities in the joint being treated and quantitation methods could be used before and after therapy. History of arthroscopy must be checked. Ultrasound or MRI is also helpful to assess the amount of effusion, joint space, and the status of the synovium to ensure homogenous distribution of the radiopharmaceutical. Complete blood cell count must be obtained before therapy as well as pregnancy test for women of child-bearing age. Injection should be done using aseptic technique. Radiosynovectomy can generally be repeated in 6 months.

Most of the patients treated are those with rheumatoid arthritis and hemophilia. Good results are generally obtained among those patients as well as those with psoriatic arthropathy. On the other hand, in osteoarthritis with recurrent joint effusion radiosynovectomy has not been as successful in relieving the symptoms. Good response is reported in 40–70% of patients. In patients with advanced cartilage destruction or bone-on-bone interaction, the synovial membrane is likely to be practically nonexistent. Accordingly, patients with less radiological damage generally show better results than those with more severe damage. If there is initially a poor response or a relapse, more than half the patients may benefit from a reinjection.

11.9
Peptide Receptor Radionuclide Therapy

Since cells express on their plasma membranes, receptor proteins with high affinity for regulatory peptides such as somatostatin, peptide analogues are used to image and treat receptor-positive tumors. The amount of these receptors changes with diseases. Overexpression of such receptors is the pathophysiologic basis of visualization and treatment of receptor-positive tumors.

High level of expression of somatostatin receptors on several tumor cells is the molecular basis of the utilization of radiolabeled somatostatin analogues in diagnostic and therapeutic nuclear oncology. Since peptides can be produced easily, have rapid clearance, rapid tissue penetration, and low antigenicity, several labeled peptides have been developed over the last few years. These include somatostatin, cholecystokinin (CCK), gastrin, vasoactive intestinal peptide (VIP), bombesin, substance P, and neuropeptide Y (NPY) analogues has shown that In-111 DTPA octreotide effect is dependent on tumor size in animal model bearing somatostatin pancreatic tumor expressing somatostatin receptor type2 (sst_2).

Complete response was seen in 50% of tumors of 1 cm or less in diameter while the response was less pronounced with increasing tumor size. This study indicates that this therapy may be preferred to start as early as possible when tumors are small.

Yttrium-90 DOTA octreotide and lanreotide can be of benefit in certain tumors:

1. Iodine-negative metastases of differentiated thyroid cancer may express somatostatin receptors and could benefit from Y-90 DOTA octreotide or lanreotide. Detection of somatostatin-positive metastases before considering this treatment should be done using diagnostic In-111 octreotide or lanreotide. Some metastases respond to octreotide while others respond to lanreotide, and there is no apparent explanation. Combination of I-131 and Y-90 DOTA octreotide or lanreotide is being considered.
2. Treatment of endocrine gastropancreatic (GEP) tumors which express somatostatin receptors.

Holmium-166 tetraphosphate (Ho-166 DOTMP), a high-energy beta emitter, is now used in treating bone and bone marrow-based tumors such as multiple myeloma. The mechanism of action is through cell death by beta particles.

11.10
Treatment of Hepatocellular Carcinoma and Liver Metastases

Blood supply to the normal liver depends on portal vein and to a much lesser extent on hepatic artery. Tumors on the other hand depend for their blood supply on arterial supply and are additionally hypervascular. This forms the basis of intraarterial therapy for hepatocellular carcinomas as well as metastatic foci. Ho-166 chitosan, Ho-166 Microspheres, Re-188 microspheres, Re-188 lipiodol, and Y-90 microspheres are all being used. This therapy is used as an adjunct therapy before and after surgery and it may be curative. Combined I-131 lipiodol and chemotherapy is also being studied.

11.11
Summary

Radionuclide therapy is effective, safe, and cost effective, and deserves consideration earlier in the management of cancer patients rather than being left as a terminal choice. Several radiopharmaceuticals are being used with varying degrees of success in treating several benign and malignant disease processes. More choices in radionuclide therapy are now available to the physicians for local and systemic uses to palliation and definitive therapy. Clinical acceptance is expected to increase as oncologists accept more the limitations of the curative and palliative role of chemotherapy and external radiation. In addition to malignant tumors, radionuclide therapy is useful in certain benign conditions such as hyperthyroidism and joint disease. The areas of research in the field of therapeutic nuclear medicine are wide open for developing new therapeutic radiopharmaceuticals and clinical applications.

Further Reading

Brans B, Bacher K, Vandevyver V, Vanlangenhove P, Smeets P, Thierens H, Dierckx RA et al (2003) Intra-arterial radionuclide therapy for liver tumors: effect of selectivity of catheterization and 131I-Lipiodol delivery on tumor uptake and response. Nucl Med Commun 24:391–396

Elgazzar AH (2006) Therapeutic nuclear medicine. In: Elgazzar AH (ed) Pathophysiologic basis of nuclear medicine, 2nd edn. Springer, Berlin

Iagaru A, McDougall IR (2007) Treatment of thyrotoxicosis. J Nucl Med 48:379–389

Mothersill C et al (2006) Targeted radiotherapy: is the "holy grail" in sight? J Nucl Med 47:27N–27N

Shankar LK et al (2006) Consensus recommendations for the use of F-18 FDG PET as an indicator of therapeutic response in patients in national cancer institute trials. J Nucl Med 47: 1059–1066

Glossary

Abscess A collection of pus in tissues, organs, or confined spaces, usually caused by bacterial infection.

Absorbed dose Amount of energy absorbed per unit mass of target material.

Antibody A protein formed by the body to defend it against disease such as infection as well as others.

Attenuation The reduction of radiation intensity during its passage through matter due to absorption, scatter, or both.

Complex Regional Pain Syndrome type I (Reflex sympathetic dystrophy) A pain syndrome that usually develops after an initiating noxious event with no identifiable major nerve injury, is not limited to the distribution of a single peripheral nerve, and is disproportional to the inciting event or expected healing response.

Cushing's disease A disease caused by abnormal stimulation of zona fasciculata of adrenal gland leading to excessive secretion of cortisol. The stimulation of the zona fasciculata may be stimulated by excess ACTH from the pituitary gland, or less commonly, the ectopic production of ACTH (as in small cell lung cancer and neural crest tumors) or corticotropin-releasing factor (as in bronchial carcinoid and prostate cancer). The disease may also be due to autonomous adrenal cortisol production due to adrenal adenoma, or hyperfunctioning adrenal carcinoma.

Dosimetry A process of calculating the level of radiation exposure from a radioactive source.

Epididymitis An inflammotory condition affecting the epididymis usually in adults secondary to infection or following trauma. Bacteria usually reach the epididymis from the prostate, seminal vesicles, urethra, or uncommonly hematogenous.

Fibrous dysplasia A benign bone disorder characterized by the presence in the fibrous tissue in lesions of trabeculae of non-lamellar bone (woven bone) which remains essentially unchanged.

A.H. Elgazzar, *A Concise Guide to Nuclear Medicine*,
DOI: 10.1007/978-3-642-19426-9, © Springer-Verlag Berlin Heidelberg 2011

Heterotopic ossification A specific type of soft tissue calcification that may or may not follow trauma and is due to a complex pathogenetic mechanism believed to be due to transformation of certain primitive cells of mesenchymal origin in the connective tissue septa within muscles, into bone-forming cells.

Hibernated myocardium Hibernation occurs in myocardium that has undergone a down-regulation of contractile function, thus reducing cellular demand for energy, in response to chronic ischemia. It requires the restoration of blood flow in order to improve function.

Hydrocephalus Describes conditions that produce imbalance between the rate of production and absorption of the cerebrospinal fluid, leading to dilatation of the ventricular system. It may result from obstruction to the flow and absorption of CSF or rarely from overproduction of CSF.

Inflammation A complex nonspecific tissue reaction to injury such as living agents as bacteria and viruses leading to infection, or nonliving agents including chemical, physical, immunologic, or radiation injurious agents.

Inflammatory bowel disease (IBD) Is an idiopathic disease, probably involving an immune reaction of the body to its own intestinal tract. The two major types of IBDs are ulcerative colitis and Crohn's disease.

Inonizing radiation A radiation that causes ionization (production of ion pair) when passing through a material.

Lisfranc injury Fracture or fracture-dislocation of tarsometatarsal joints.

Monoclonal antibody An antibody derived from a single clone of cells and hence binds only to one unique epitope.

Neuroblastoma A malignant tumor of the sympathetic nervous system of childhood. It accounts for up to 10% of childhood cancers and 15% of cancer deaths among children. Seventy-five percent of neuroblastoma patients are younger than 4 years. The tumor has the potential to mature into pheochromocytoma or ganglioneuroma.

Osteomalacia Abnormal mineralization of bone with a decrease in bone density secondary to lack of both calcium and phosphorus with no decrease in the amount of osteoid (bone formation).

Osteomyelitis A term applied to skeletal infection when it involves the bone marrow.

Osteoporosis Reduction of bone tissue amount increasing the likelihood of fractures.

Pheochromocytoma A rare tumor arising from chromaffin cells of the adrenal medulla. It commonly produces excessive amounts of norepinephrine, attributable to autonomous functioning of the tumor, although large tumors secrete both norepinephrine and epinephrine and in some cases also dopamine. Releasing the catecholamine into the circulation causes hypertension and other signs.

Physical half-life Time required for half of a radioactivity to decay.

Pneumocystis carinii (jiroveci) An opportunistic pathogen currently classified as a fungus. It causes infection leading to significant morbidity and mortality in human immunodeficiency virus–associated and nonhuman immunodeficiency virus–associated immunosuppressed patients, although it also occurs in nonimmunocompromised patients.

Radionuclide synovectomy Destruction of the diseases synovial membrane by radiopharmaceuticals when injected intraarticularly to relive pain.

Renal osteodystrophy A metabolic condition of bone associated with chronic renal failure.

Sarcoidosis A multisystem granulomatous disorder, occurs most commonly in young adults, more commonly in blacks and in temperate areas with unknown etiology, but it is believed to be due to exaggerated cellular immune response on the part of helper/inducer T lymphocytes to exogenous or autoantigens.

Sentinel lymph node Is the hypothetical first lymph node or group of nodes reached by metastasizing cancer cells from a primary tumor.

Spondylolysis A loss of continuity of bone of the neuroarch of the vertebra due to stress or trauma.

Stress fracture A pathologic real high turn over condition of bone due to repeated episodes of stress, each is less forceful than that needed to cause acute fracture of the bony cortex.

Stunned myocardium Continued dysfunction due to ischemia-induced oxidative stress.

Woven bone Immature non-lamellar bone that is later normally converted to lamellar bone.

Index

A.H. Elgazzar, *A Concise Guide to Nuclear Medicine,*
DOI: 10.1007/978-3-642-19426-9, © Springer-Verlag Berlin Heidelberg 2011

Printing: Ten Brink, Meppel, The Netherlands
Binding: Stürtz, Würzburg, Germany